Moshe Schein

Schein's Common Sense Emergency Abdominal Surgery

Springer

Berlin
Heidelberg
New York
Barcelona
Hong Kong
London
Milan
Paris
Singapore
Tokyo

Moshe Schein

Schein's Common Sense Emergency Abdominal Surgery

A Small Book for Residents, Thinking Surgeons and Even Students

With contributions by:

Adam Klipfel, MD, Assistant Editor (USA)
Bashar H. Fahoum, MD, FACS (USA)
Gary Gecelter, MD, FACS (USA)
Pioter Gorecki, MD (USA)
Asher Hirshberg, MD (USA)
Per-Olof Nyström, MD (Sweden)
Paul Rogers, FRCS (Scotland)
James C. Rucinski, MD, FACS (USA)
Roger Saadia, MD, FRCS (Canada)

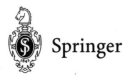 Springer

Moshe Schein, MD, FACS, FCS (SA)
Associate Professor of Surgery
Cornell University Medical College, NY,
Attending Surgeon,
New York Methodist Hospital,
506 Sixth Street
11215-9008 Brooklyn, NY, USA

ISBN 3-540-66654-0 Springer-Verlag Berlin Heidelberg New York

CIP data applied for
Schein, Moshe:
Schein's common sense emergency abdominal surgery : a small book for residents,
thinking surgeons and even students / Moshe Schein. With contributions by:
B. H. Fahoum .... - Berlin ; Heidelberg ; New York ; Barcelona ; Hong Kong ; London ;
Milan ; Paris ; Singapore ; Tokyo :
Springer, 2000
  ISBN 3-540-66654-0

Springer-Verlag is a company in the BertelsmannSpringer publishing group.
© Springer-Verlag Berlin Heidelberg 2000
Printed in Italy

The use of general descriptive names, registered names, trademarks, etc. in this pub-
lication does not imply, even in the absence of a specific statement, that such names
are exempt from the relevant protective laws and regulations and therefore free for
general use

Product liability: The publishers cannot guarantee the accuracy of any information
about the application of operative techniques and medications contained in this
book. In every individual case the user must check such information by consulting
the relevant literature.

Data conversion by Isolde Gundermann, Heidelberg
Cover design: design & production GmbH, Heidelberg
Printed on acid-free paper   SPIN 10708197   24/3133/is   5 4 3 2 1 0

This book is dedicated to my father –
a war surgeon – on the Russian-German front
during the Second World War.

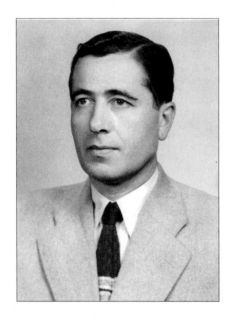

"During each later war I watched surgeons committing
the same basic errors I learned to avoid during 1940.
Such a waste in young lives..."

Karl Schein, MD (1911–1974)

Acknowledgments

This book has been assembled – in pieces – during twenty years of intensive personal involvement, clinical and academic, with emergency abdominal surgery in South Africa, Israel and the USA. For the foundations in this noble surgical field I am indebted to George G. Decker of Johannesburg. About half of the chapters were written in collaboration with my good old friends from around the world, who are listed in the list of contributors. Many thanks to Roger Saadia, Asher Hirshberg, Per-Olof Nyström, and Paul Rogers, who did not spare encouragement and sound advice. Eric Frykberg and the members of SURGINET helped find the title to this book and test-read selected chapters. Alfredo Sepulvede provided a few aphorisms and quotations. I am grateful to Adam Klipfel for proofreading the manuscript, to our surgical residents for continuously exciting my mind, to Syed Gardezi for his friendship, and my Chairman – Leslie Wise for providing me with a safe haven to pursue my interests.

Special thanks to Agnes Heinz, Ph.D., Springer Verlag, Heidelberg, for trusting me with this allegedly unconventional book. Finally, it is my loving and minimally nagging wife Heidi, and my good sons Omri, Yariv and Dan, who let me spend all those years writing-instead of making more money and entertaining them.

The reader will find that there are not a few duplications scattered along the book. We did it on purpose, as repetition of important points is crucial in adult education. Any reader who has a question or a comment about anything mentioned in this book is invited to e-mail me directly – *mschein1@mindspring.com* – I will respond.

Moshe Schein, Brooklyn
August 1999

Preface

Smart surgeons learn from their own mistakes,
smarter surgeons learn from mistakes of others,
some never learn...

You are a resident, overworked and constantly tired; sitting down with your mentor for a brief tutorial. What do you want to get out of these few minutes? To organize your thoughts and approaches to the particular problem; to learn how he – the weathered surgeon – "tackles it"; to grasp a few practical "recipes" or "goodies" and take home a message or two; to laugh a bit and unwind. This is also our goal in this book.

We hope that you are not repelled or offended by the non-formal character of this book. This is how emergency abdominal surgery is taught best, by trial and error and repetitions, with emphasis on basics. This is not a "complete" textbook, nor is it a cookbook type manual or discussion of case studies; neither is it a collection of detailed lecture notes or exhaustive lists. Instead, it consists of a series of informal, uncensored, chats between experienced surgeons and their trainees. No percentages, series, elaborated figures or complicated algorithms are included; only a surgeon's narrative, explaining how "he does it" – based on his experience and state of the art knowledge of the literature. No references are included as it was our aim to put down nothing which has not been experienced, confirmed and practiced in our own hands. The starting point of each individual contribution is that there are many ways to skin a cat, or different clinical pathways to arrive at a similar outcome; however, one of the options is *"better"*. Another emphasis was on common pitfalls and mistakes.

This book comprises of short chapters, which are allocated to three sections: preoperative phase, the operation, and postoperative phase. The chapters supplement each other and are best not read in isolation.

For the surgeon, emergency surgery has always been, and still is, what the battleground is for the soldier, an exhilarating place – a character-building source of skill, experience, excitement and glory. Emergency surgery remains the playing field where the surgical boys (girls) become men (women). Surgical trainees adhere to this myth and hence their inherent attraction to this topic. We hope that this book will increase your fascination with emergency abdominal surgery, helping you to practice it better.

Contents

Contributors

Bashar H. Fahoum, MD, FACS
Attending Surgeon, Director S.I.C.U.
Department of Surgery
New York Methodist Hospital
506 Sixth St. - 6th Fl.
Brooklyn, New York 11215, USA
(Chapter 25)

Gary Gecelter, MD, FACS
Chief, Division of General Surgery
Long Island Jewish Medical Center
270-05 76th Avenue, Research Building – Room B-235
New Hyde Park, New York 11040, USA
(Chapter 16)

Pioter Gorecki, MD
Attending Surgeon
Department of Surgery
Nassau County Hospital
2201 Hempstead Tpk.
East Meadow, New York 11554, USA
(Chapter 41)

Asher Hirshberg, MD
Associate Professor of Surgery
Department of Surgery
Baylor College of Medicine & Ben Taub General Hospital
Houston, Texas, USA
(Chapter 2, 3, 8, 9, 25, 26, 27)

Adam Klipfel, MD
Surgical Resident
Department of Surgery
New York Methodist Hospital
506 Sixth St. - 6th Fl.
Brooklyn, New York 11215, USA
(Assistant Editor)

xiv   Per-Olof Nyström, MD
      Associate Professor
      The University of Linkoping
      Chief of Colorectal Surgery
      Linkoping University Hospital
      58185 Linkoping, Sweden
      (Chapter 20, 21, 23,24)

      Paul Rogers, FRCS
      Consultant, General and Vascular Surgery
      Department of Surgery
      Gartnavel Western Hospital
      Ardersier
      59 Langlands Drive
      Newlands, Glasgow G43 2QX, Scotland
      (Chapter 3, 18)

      James C. Rucinski, MD, FRCS
      Instructor in Surgery
      Director of Surgical Education
      New York Methodist Hospital
      506 Sixth St. - 6th Fl.
      Brooklyn, New York 11215, USA
      (Chapter 5, 7, 19, 31)

      Roger Saadia, MD, FRCS
      Professor of Surgery
      Department of Surgery
      University of Manitoba
      Health Sciences Center and St Boniface General Hospital
      Winnipeg, Canada
      (Chapter 10, 17, 26, 27, 32, 33, 37)

1　General Philosophy

Surgeons are internists who operate...

Wisdom comes alone through suffering
(Aeschylus, Agamemnon).

At this moment – just when you pick up this book, beginning to browse through its pages – there are thousands of surgeons around the world facing a patient with an abdominal catastrophe. The platform on which such an encounter takes place differs from place to place – be it a modern emergency department in London, a shabby casualty room in the Bronx, or doctor's tent in an African bush – the scene itself is amazingly uniform. It is always the same: you confronting a patient. He – in pain, suffering and anxious; you anxious as well. Anxious about the diagnosis, concerned about which is the best management, troubled about your own abilities to do what is correct. We arrived at the year 2000 – but this universal scenario is not original. It is as old as modern surgery itself. You are perhaps too young to note how little things changed along the path of years. Yes, your hospital may be in the forefront of modern medicine, it's emergency room has a standby, state-of-art spiral CT and MRI machines, but practically – nothing has changed. It is the patient against you – you who are bound to provide a correct management plan and execute it.

The "Best" Management of an Abdominal Emergency

It is useful to liken the emergency abdominal surgeon to a leader of foot soldiers. Away from the limelight and glory, which surrounds cardiac or neurological surgeons, emergency abdominal surgery resembles more the infantry than the airforce. A war cannot be won in remote control by

2   cruise missiles but with infantry on the ground. Likewise, technological gimmicks have little place in emergency abdominal surgery, which is the domain of the surgeon's brain and hands. With the infantry, emergency abdominal surgery shares a few simple rules – accumulated in the trenches and during offensives – rules which are the key to victory and survival. Such code of the battle echoes the "best" management of abdominal emergencies.

	Infantry	Emergency abdominal surgery
Rule 1	Destroy your enemy before he destroys you	Save lives
Rule 2	Spare your own men	Reduce morbidity
Rule 3	Save ammunition	Use resources rationally
Rule 4	Know your enemy	Estimate severity of disease
Rule 5	Know your men	Understand the risk-benefit ratio of your therapy
Rule 6	Attack at "soft" points	Tailor your management to the disease and the patient
Rule 7	Do not call for airforce support in a hand-to-hand battle	Do not adopt useless gimmicks – use your mind and hands
Rule 8	Conduct the battle from the line of fire – not from the rear	Do not take and accept decisions over the phone
Rule 9	Take advice from the generals but the decision is yours	Procure and use consultation from "other specialties" selectively
Rule 10	Maintain high moral among your troops	Be proud in providing the "best" management

From your previous or current surgical mentors you know that there are many ways to skin a cat and different clinical pathways to arrive at a similar outcome. However, only one of the diverse pathways is the "correct one" – thus – the *"best!"*. To be considered as such the "preferred pathway" has to save life and decrease morbidity in the most efficient way. Look at this example: you can manage perforated acute appendicitis

using two different pathways – both leading to an eventual recovery and
both considered absolutely appropriate.

Pathway 1	Pathway 2
Young male – right lower quadrant peritonitis	Young male – right lower quadrant peritonitis
***	CT scan
Appendectomy for gangrenous appendicitis – 3 hours after admission	Appendectomy for gangrenous appendicitis – 36 hours after admission
Primary closure of the wound	Wound left open
24 hours of postoperative antibiotics	Five days of postoperative antibiotics
***	Secondary closure of wound
Discharge home on the third postoperative day	Discharge home on the seventh postoperative day

Both above pathways are OK, right? Yes, but pathway 1 clearly is the "best" one.

Today many options exist to do almost anything. Just clicking-open the
MEDLINE you are overwhelmed with numerous papers, which can prove
and justify almost anything you elect to do. Data and theory are everywhere – the sources are numerous but what you really need is *wisdom* to
enable you to correctly apply the knowledge you already have and are
surrounded with.

General Philosophy

"There is nothing new in the story..." Winston Churchill said, "want of
foresight, unwillingness to act when action would be simple and effective,
lack of clear thinking, confusion of counsel until the emergency comes,
until self preservation strikes its jarring gong...". How true is this
Chuchillian wisdom when applied to emergency surgery. How often we
forget old – written in stone – principles while re-inventing the wheel?

4   The "best" management in each section of this book is based on the following elements:
- Old – established principles (not to re-invent the wheel).
- Modern – scientific understanding of inflammation and infection.
- Evidence based surgery (see below).
- Personal experience.

The Inflamed Patient

Think about your patient as being INFLAMED by a myriad of inflammatory mediators, generated by the primary disease process, be it inflammatory, infectious or traumatic. That local (e. g. peritonitis) and systemic inflammation (SIRS) are the ones that lead to organ dysfunction or failure, and the eventual demise of your patient. The greater is the inflammation, the sicker is the patient, and higher is the expected mortality and morbidity. Think also that anything you do to halt your patient's inflammation may in fact contribute to it – adding wood into the inflammatory fire. Too big an operation, inappropriately performed, and too late, just adds nails onto your patients' coffin. The philosophy of treatment that we wish to bestow upon you maintains that in order to effectively cure or minimize the inflammatory processes the management should be accurately tailored to the individual patient's disease. The punishment should fit the crime-there is no use to indiscriminately fire at all directions!

Evidence

A few words about what we mean when we talk about "evidence".

Evidence level	Description	5
I	A scientifically sound RCT*	
II	RCT with methodological "problems"	
III	Non-randomized concurrent cohort comparison	
IV	Non-randomized historical cohort comparison	
V	A case series without controls	

To the above "official" classification we wish to add another three categories frequently used by surgeons around the world:

VI	"In my personal series of X patients (never published) there were no complications"
VII	"I remember that case..."
VIII	"This is the way I do it and it is the best"

* RCT- randomized controlled trial

Note that level V studies form the main bulk of surgical literature, which deals with abdominal emergencies, whereas level VI-VIII evidence is the main form of evidence used by surgeons in general. You should educate yourself to think in terms of levels of evidence. As usual – when high level of evidence is not available – we have to use an individual approach and common sense – which will be herein emphasized.

You can get away with a lot...but not always. Most patients treated according to the above mentioned pathway #2 will do well but a few will not. The following pages will help you to develop your own judgement – pointing to the correct pathway in any situation. This is obviously not a Bible but it is based on a thorough knowledge of the literature and a vast personal experience. So wherever you are – in Pakistan, Norway, Chile' or Canada and whatever are your resources – the approach to emergency abdominal surgery is the same: come and join us – to save lives, decrease morbidity – and do it correctly!

The operation is a silent confession to the surgeon's inadequacy (John Hunter)

Section A:

Before the Operation

2   The Acute Abdomen

For the abdominal surgeon it is a familiar experience to sit,
ready scrubbed and gowned, in a corner of the quiet theatre,
with the clock pointing midnight....

In a few minutes the patient will be wheeled in
and another emergency laparotomy will commence.
This is the culmination of a process
which begun a few hours previously
with the surgeon meeting with
and examining the patient,
reaching a diagnosis,
and making a plan of action.
(Peter F. Jones)

Simply stated, the term acute abdomen refers to abdominal pain of short
duration that requires a decision regarding whether an urgent operation
is necessary. This clinical problem is the most common cause for you to
be called to provide a surgical consultation in the emergency room
and serves as a convenient gateway for a discussion of the approach to
abdominal surgical emergencies.

The Problem

Most major textbooks contain a long list of possible causes for acute
abdominal pain, often enumerating 20-30 "most common" etiologies.
These "big lists" usually go from perforated peptic ulcer down to such
esoteric causes as porphyria and black widow spider bites. The lists are
popular with medical students, but totally useless for practical guys like
you.

10   The experienced surgical resident called upon to consult a patient
with acute abdominal pain in the emergency room (ER) in the middle of
the night simply does not work this way. He or she does not consider the
fifty or so "most likely" causes of acute abdominal pain from the list and
does not attempt to rule them out one by one. Instead, the smart surgical
resident tries to identify a *clinical pattern*, and to decide upon a course
of action from a limited menu of options. Below we will demonstrate
how the multiple etiologies for acute abdominal pain actually converge
into a small number of easily recognizable clinical patterns. Once
recognized, each of these patterns dictates a specific course of action.

The Management Options

Seeing a patient with an acute abdomen in the ER you have only four
possible management options:
- Immediate operation ("surgery now").
- Pre-operative preparation and operation ("surgery tonight").
- Conservative treatment (active observation, IV fluids, antibiotics, etc.)
- Discharge home.

The last option (discharge) deserves some consideration. Many patients
with acute abdominal pain undergo a clinical examination and a limited
workup only to be labeled as *"non-specific abdominal pain"* (NSAP) and
then discharged. NSAP is a clinical entity albeit an ill-defined one. It is a
type of acute abdominal pain that is severe enough to bring a patient to
seek medical attention. The patient's physical examination and diagnostic
work-up are negative, and the pain is self-limited and usually does not
recur. It is important to keep in mind that in an ER setting, more than
half the patients presenting with acute abdominal pain have NSAP, with
acute appendicitis and acute cholecystitis the commonest "specific"

conditions. But the exact pathology you see depends of course on your geographical location and pattern of practice. Just remember that patients discharged home labeled with the diagnosis of NSAP have a higher probability to be diagnosed subsequently with an abdominal cancer. Therefore, referral for elective investigations may be indicated

The Clinical Patterns

The acute abdomen presents as one of five distinct and well-defined clinical patterns:
- Abdominal pain and shock
- Generalized peritonitis
- Localized peritonitis (confined to one quadrant of the abdomen)
- Intestinal obstruction
- Important medical causes

Two additional patterns (trauma and gynecological problems) are addressed elsewhere in this volume.

Each of these clinical patterns dictates a specific management option. Thus it is sufficient to identify the pattern to know what needs to be done with the patient.

Abdominal Pain and Shock

This is the most dramatic and least common clinical pattern of the acute abdomen. The patient typically presents pale and diaphoretic, in severe abdominal pain and with hypotension, the so-called "abdominal apoplexy". The two most common etiologies of this clinical pattern are a ruptured *abdominal aortic aneurysm* and a ruptured *ectopic pregnancy* (chapters 30 & 25). The only management option is an immediate *"surgery-now"*.

12 No time should be wasted on "preparations" and on ancillary investigations. Losing a patient with abdominal apoplexy in the CT scanner is a cardinal, and unfortunately not too rare, sin.

Generalized Peritonitis

The clinical picture of generalized peritonitis consists of diffuse severe abdominal pain in a patient who looks sick and toxic. The patient typically lies motionless, and has an extremely tender abdomen with "peritoneal signs" consisting of board-like rigidity, rebound-tenderness, and voluntary defense-guarding. Surprisingly enough, less experienced clinicians occasionally miss the diagnosis entirely. This is especially common in the geriatric patient who may have weak abdominal musculature or may not exhibit the classical peritoneal signs. The most common error in the physical examination of a patient with acute abdominal pain is rough and „deep" palpation of the abdomen, which may elicit severe tenderness even in a patient without any abdominal pathology. Palpation of the abdomen should be very gentle, and should not hurt the patient. The umbilicus is the shallowest part of the abdominal wall where the peritoneum almost touches the skin. Thus one of the most effective maneuvers in the physical examination of a patient suspected of having peritonitis is gentle palpation in the umbilical groove, where tenderness is very obvious. We appreciate that at this stage of your surgical career you do not need a detailed lecture on the examination of the acute abdomen. Forgive us, however, for emphasizing that the absence of rebound tenderness means nothing and that a good way to elicit peritoneal irritation is by asking the patient to cough, shaking (gently) his bed, and with very gentle percussion of the abdomen.

The two most common causes of generalized peritonitis in adults are a *perforated ulcer* (chapter 13) and a *colonic perforation* (chapter 23) (In the pediatric age group, perforated appendicitis is the most common

cause (chapter 22). The management of a patient with diffuse peritonitis   13
is pre-operative preparation and operation *("surgery tonight")*. The
patient should be taken to the operating room only after adequate pre-
operative preparation as outlined in chapter 5.

The only important exception to this management option is the
patient with *acute pancreatitis*. While most patients with acute pancreatitis
present with mild epigastric tenderness, the occasional patient may
present with a clinical picture mimicking diffuse peritonitis (chapter 14).
As a precaution against missing these patients, it is good practice to
always obtain serum amylase in any patient presenting with significant
abdominal symptoms (chapter 3).

Localized Peritonitis

In the patient with localized peritonitis, the clinical signs are confined to
one quadrant of the abdomen. In the RLQ the most common cause of
localized peritonitis is *acute appendicitis* (chapter 22). In the RUQ it is
acute cholecystitis (chapter 15), and in the LLQ it is *acute diverticulitis*
(chapter 23). Peritonitis confined to the LUQ is uncommon.

As a general rule, localized peritonitis is not always an indication for a
"surgery tonight" policy. Instead, when diagnosis is uncertain it may be
initially treated conservatively. The patient is admitted to the surgical
floor, given IV antibiotics (if the diagnosis of acute cholecystitis or
diverticulitis – for example – is entertained) and hydration, and is
actively observed by means of serial physical exams. *Time is a superb
diagnostician*: when you return to the patient's bedside after a few
hours – you may find all the previously missing clues.

The only universal exception to this rule is of course a tender RLQ,
where the working diagnosis is acute appendicitis, and appendectomy is
therefore clearly indicated. However, if there is a palpable mass in the

RLQ, the working diagnosis is a "appendiceal phlegmon" for which an appropriate initial management would be conservative (chapter 22).

The management of *acute cholecystitis* varies among surgeons. While it is usually safe to treat these patients initially with antibiotics, most surgeons elect to operate on a "hot" gallbladder. This policy of "same night" surgery or "surgery in the morning" is certainly justified in any patient whose cholecystitis worsens under the conservative regimen, in the elderly diabetic and in immuno-compromised patients where the gallbladder inflammation is unlikely to settle on antibiotics alone (chapter 15).

Intestinal Obstruction

The clinical picture of intestinal obstruction consists of central, colicky abdominal pain, distention, constipation and vomiting. Vomiting and colicky pain are more characteristic of *small bowel obstruction* while constipation and gross distention is typical of *colonic obstruction*. However, the distinction between these two kinds of obstruction usually hinges on the plain abdominal X-ray. There are two management options for these patients: conservative treatment and operative treatment after adequate preparation. The major problem with intestinal obstruction is not in making the diagnosis but in deciding on the appropriate course of action. If the patient has a history of previous abdominal surgery and presents with small bowel obstruction but without signs of peritonitis, the working diagnosis is "simple" adhesive small bowel obstruction. The initial management of these patients is conservative, with IV fluids and nasogastric tube decompression. If the obstruction is complete (i.e. no gas in the colon above the peritoneal reflection of the rectum), the chances of spontaneous resolution are small and some surgeons would opt for an operative intervention. In the presence of a tender abdomen, fever, or a progressively elevated WBC count, the indication for laparotomy is clear-cut (see chapter 17).

There are three *classical pitfalls* with small bowel obstruction:

- The obese elderly lady with no previous surgical history who presents with small bowel obstruction, where an incarcerated femoral hernia can easily be missed if not specifically sought.
- The elderly patient with a "simple" adhesive small bowel obstruction who improves on conservative treatment and is discharged only to later come back with a large tumor mass in the right colon.
- The patient with a history of previous gastric surgery who presents with intermittent episodes of obstruction originating from a bezoar in the terminal ileum.

Unlike small bowel obstruction, colon obstruction is always an indication for surgery – "tonight or tomorrow" but usually "tomorrow". The diagnosis cannot be made by a plain abdominal X-ray where functional *pseudocolonic obstruction* (Ogilvie's syndrome) or chronic megacolon cannot be reliably distinguished from a mechanical obstruction. Thus these patients usually undergo either fibro-optic sigmoidoscopy or a contrast enema to clinch the diagnosis. The management option for these patients is operation after adequate preparation (chapter 21).

Important Medical Causes

While there is a large number of non-surgical causes that may result in acute abdominal pain, two must be constantly kept in your mind: *inferior wall MI* and *diabetic ketoacidosis*. A negative laparotomy for porphyria or even basal pneumonia is an unfortunate surgical (and medico-legal) occurrence, but inadvertently operating on a patient with an undiagnosed inferior wall MI or diabetic ketoacidosis may well be a lethal mistake that should be avoided at all costs.

16   Conclusion

The multiple etiologies of the acute abdomen converge to five distinct
and well – defined clinical patterns, each of which is associated with
a specific management option. You should be familiar with the patterns
and with the management options, and should also keep in mind the
classical pitfalls inherent in this common surgical condition in order to
avoid gross errors in the surgical care of these patients. You already have
enough cases to present at the M & M Meeting, don't you? (chapter 42).

> **It is as much an intellectual exercise to tackle the problems
> of belly ache as to work on the human genome
> (Hugh Dudley)**

3   Rational Diagnostic Procedures

Believe nobody – question everything

When treating a patient with acute abdominal pain it is tempting to make extensive use of ancillary investigations. This leads to the emergence of "routines" in the emergency room (ER) whereby every patient with acute abdominal pain undergoes a plain X-ray of the abdomen (AXR) and a series of blood tests which typically include a complete blood count, routine blood chemistry and serum amylase. These "routine" tests have a very low diagnostic yield and are not cost-effective. However, they are also an unavoidable part of life in the ER and are usually obtained before the surgical consultation.

For the patient who on examination has a clear-cut *diffuse peritonitis* no imaging is necessary because a laparotomy is indicated. But what appears clear cut to the experienced surgeon may be less so for you. Bear in mind the following caveats:

- *Intestinal distension*, associated with obstruction or inflammation (e.g., enteritis or colitis) may produce diffuse abdominal tenderness – mimicking "peritonitis" – the "whole" clinical picture as well as the AXR will guide you toward the proper diagnosis. (chapters 17 & 21)
- *Acute pancreatitis* may present with clinical acute peritonitis. You should obtain, therefore, a serum *amylase* level in order to avoid falling in the not so uncommon trap of unnecessarily operating on acute pancreatitis. (chapter 14)
- In any patient who receives or has recently received any quantity of antibiotics think about *C. difficile entero-colitis* which may present – from the beginning – as an acute abdomen without diarrhea. Here, the optimal initial management is medical and not a laparotomy; bedside sigmoidoscopy and/or CT may be diagnostic. (chapter 21)

18   Chest X-Ray (CXR)

A CXR is routinely obtained to search for free air under the diaphragms which is demonstrated in the majority of patients with perforated peptic ulcer (chapter 13) but less frequently when colonic perforation is the underlying problem (chapter 23). Remember that free air is better seen on CXR than AXR. Free intra-peritoneal air is not always caused by a perforated viscus and it is not always an indication for a laparotomy. There is a long list of "non-operative" conditions, which may produce free intra-peritoneal air such as a tension pneumothorax or even vigorous felatio (oral sex). So do not be dogmatic and look at the whole clinical picture.

Any text book tells you that lower lobe pneumonia may mimic an "acute abdomen" so think about it. Obviously, findings such as lung metastases or pleural effusion may hint to the cause of the abdominal condition and influence treatment and prognosis. Pneumothorax, pnenumomediastinum or pleural effusion may be associated with spontaneous esophageal perforation (Boerhaave's syndrome) which can present as an acute abdomen. The value of a CXR in blunt or penetrating abdominal injury is obvious. A pre-operative CXR is also requested by the anesthesiologists, especially after you have inserted a central venous line.

Plain Abdominal X-Ray (AXR)

This is the classical surgeon's X-ray as only surgeons know how to rely on those simple and cheap radiographs. Radiologists can look and talk about AXR's forever, searching for findings which could justify "additional" imaging studies. We, surgeons need only a few seconds to decide whether the AXR is *"non-specific"*, namely, does not show any obvious abnormality, or one of the following is present: *abnormal gas pattern or abnormal "opacities."*

Abnormal Gas Pattern

- *Free air* was discussed above. If CXR is "normal" and you suspect a perforation of a viscus, a right lateral decubitus abdominal film may show free air in the peritoneal cavity. Make a habit to always look for atypical free air patterns – occasionally it may reward you with an eye-popping diagnosis: air in the bile ducts implies a cholecysto-enteric fistula (gallstone ileus – chapter 17) or status post sphincterotomy of the sphincter of Oddi. Air within the wall of gallbladder signifies a necrotizing infection (chapter 15). *Soap-bubble appearance* signifies free air in the *retroperitoneum*: in the epigastrium it is associated with *infected pancreatic necrosis* (chapter 14), in the right upper quadrant with a retroperitoneal perforation of the duodenum, and in the gutters – with retroperitoneal perforation of the colon.
- Abnormal gaseous distension/dilatation of *small bowel*, with or without air/fluid levels, implies a small bowel process – be it *obstructive* (small bowel obstruction – chapter 17), *paralytic* (ileus – chapter 34) or *inflammatory* (Crohn's – chapter 20). Remember – *acute gastroenteritis* may produce small bowel air/fluid levels: the diarrhea hints to the diagnosis.
- Abnormal gaseous distension/dilatation of the *colon* denotes colonic *obstruction or volvulus* (chapter 21), colonic *inflammation* (inflammatory bowel disease – chapter 20) or colonic ileus (pseudo-obstruction – chapter 21).

Distinguishing small bowel from colon on AXR is easy: the "transverse lines" cross the whole circumference of the small bowel (the valvulae conniventes) and only a portion of the circumference of the colon (the haustra).

Useful Rules of Thumb

- Gaseous distension of small bowel + no air in the colon = complete small bowel obstruction
- Significant gaseous distension of small bowel + minimal quantity of colonic air = partial small bowel obstruction
- Significant gaseous distension of both the small bowel and the colon = paralytic ileus
- Significant gaseous distension of the colon + minimal distention of the small bowel = colonic obstruction or pseudo-obstruction

Abnormal Opacities

The opacities which you are able to spot on AXR are the calcified ones: gallstones – visible in about one third of cases, ureteric stones visible in most patients with renal colic, pancreatic calcifications in some patients with chronic pancreatitis, and appendicular fecaliths, occasionally seen in patients with perforated appendicitis.

Fecal matter may opacify the rectum and colon to a various degree – achieving extreme proportions in patients with fecal impaction.

Abdominal Ultrasound (US)

Abdominal US is a readily available diagnostic modality in most places. Its reliability is operator dependent; the ideal situation is when the US is performed and interpreted by an experienced clinician – a surgeon. US is very accurate in the diagnosis of acute cholecystitis (chapter 15); it is also used by the gynecologists to rule out acute pelvic pathology in female patients (chapter 25), and to demonstrate an acutely obstructed kidney caused by a ureteric stone. A non-compressible tubular structure

(a "small sausage") in the right lower quadrant may be diagnostic of acute
appendicitis, but as discussed in chapter 22 you rarely need abdominal
imaging to reach this diagnosis. US is useful in demonstrating intra-abdominal fluid – be it ascites, pus, or blood, localized or diffuse. In blunt
abdominal trauma it is emerging as a serious contender to diagnostic
peritoneal lavage (chapter 27).

Abdominal Computed Tomography (CT)

The use of the CT scan in the acute abdomen is not well defined, and
remains a subject of some controversy. While it is true that a CT scan is
not part of the management algorithm of the great majority of patients
with acute abdominal pain, the new – spiral CT technology is nevertheless
immediately available, very powerful and thus extremely tempting to use,
especially by less experienced clinicians.

A case in point is acute diverticulitis (chapter 23). Once the clinical
pattern of localized peritonitis in the LLQ has been identified, initial
management is conservative. A CT may show the inflammatory process
and even a para-colic abscess, but will not distinguish between diverticulitis and a localized perforation of a colonic tumor. In any case, this
will not alter the approach because most surgeons would still opt for
a trial of IV antibiotics as the initial treatment modality for this clinical
pattern (chapter 23).

The true role of the CT, where it can really make a critical difference,
is with "clinical puzzles". Not infrequently, the surgeon encounters a
patient with acute abdominal pain, which does not fit any of the clinical
patterns described in the previous chapter. The patient is obviously sick,
but the diagnosis remains elusive. Occasionally, there may be a suspicion
of acute intra-abdominal pathology in an unconscious patient. Under
these unusual circumstances, the CT scan may be very helpful in identi-
fying an intra-abdominal problem. It is even better in *excluding* the

latter by an absolutely normal CT. CT is frequently indicated in patients with blunt abdominal trauma as discussed below (chapter 27). Its selective use in other circumstances is dealt with in the individual chapters. CT has a definite role in the post-laparotomy patient as discussed in chapter 35.

A Word of Caution

For most patients with acute abdominal pain, unnecessary ancillary investigations are merely a resource problem and a waste of time. But for two types of surgical problems, unnecessary imaging is often lethal:

- *Acute mesenteric ischemia* is the only life-threatening abdominal condition that cannot be easily classified into one of the five clinical patterns described in chapter 2. Because of this, and because the window of opportunity to salvage viable bowel is so narrow, it behooves on you to have this diagnosis constantly embedded in the back of your mind. The best chance to salvage these patients is to identify the clinical picture of very severe abdominal pain with few objective findings in the appropriate clinical context (chapter 19) and to proceed directly to mesenteric *angiography*. Needless to say, if the patient has diffuse peritonitis, no imaging is necessary and the next step is an urgent laparotomy. The most tragic error in these patients is the inability of even an experienced clinician to make his or her mind up regarding the need for urgent angiography. As a result the patient is sent for a long series of non-relevant imaging studies and the opportunity to salvage viable bowel is lost.
- The second condition where the abuse of imaging is often lethal is with a *ruptured abdominal aortic aneurysm (AAA)* (chapter 30). A ruptured AAA may not present as abdominal pain and shock but merely as severe abdominal or back pain, and it may not be easily palpable in an obese patient. When the possibility of a

contained rupture is raised in a hemodynamically stable patient,   23
the one and only ancillary investigation that is required is an
urgent CT scan of the abdomen. Unfortunately, too many times
these patients spend several hours in the ER, waiting for the results
of non-relevant blood tests and progressing slowly along the
imaging path from AXR's – which are usually non-diagnostic – to
US – which shows the aneurysm but often cannot diagnose a rupture, to a long wait for unnecessary contrast material to fill the
bowel in preparation for a "technically perfect" CT scan. The tragic
end of these delays is a dramatic hemodynamic collapse either
before or during an abdominal CT scan.

Barium vs. Water Soluble Contrast

A caveat: in emergency situations do not use barium! Radiologists prefer
barium because of its superior imaging qualities; but for us – surgeons –
barium is an enemy. Bacteria love barium – for it protects them from the
peritoneal macrophages: a mixture of barium with feces is the best
recipe to produce intractable peritonitis and multiple intra-abdominal
abscesses. Once barium leaks into the peritoneal cavity it is very difficult
to get rid off. Barium given into the bowel from above or below tends to
stay there for many days – making a subsequent CT or arteriography
impossible to obtain.

A contrast study in the emergency situation has only two queries
to answer:
- Is there a *leak* and where?
- Is there an *obstruction* and where?

For this purpose gastrografin is adequate. Use gastrografin upper
gastrointestinal study to document or exclude gastric outlet obstruction
or a gastrografin enema to diagnose colonic obstruction or perforation.

24   Unlike barium, gastrografin is harmless should it extravasate into the peritoneal cavity. Try to operate on a colon full of barium: a clamp slides off, a stapler misfires and you – not the radiologist – are the one left to clean the mess. A sincere advice from our bitter experience: *ordering* a gastrografin study is not enough; you must personally ensure that barium is not used.

Blood Tests

As stated above "routine labs" are of minimal value. In addition to amylase level the only "routines" which can be supported are white cell count and hematocrit. *Elevated white cell count* denotes an inflammatory response to whatever cause. Be aware that you can diagnose acute chole-cystitis or acute appendicitis even when the white cell count is within a normal range. Its elevation, however, supports the diagnosis. Low *hematocrit* in the emergency situation signifies a chronic or subacute anemia, poorly reflecting on the magnitude of the acute hemorrhage. *Liver functions* are of some value in the patients with right upper quadrant pain, diagnosed to have acute cholecystitis (chapter 15) or cholangitis (chapter 16).

Whichever tests you order, or someone – usually the ER doctor – orders for you, be aware that the significance of the results should be never judged in isolation but taken together with the whole clinical picture.

Unnecessary Tests

Unnecessary testing is plaguing modern medical practice. Look around you and notice that the majority of investigations being ordered do not add much to the quality of care. Unnecessary tests, on the other hand, are expensive and potentially harmful. In addition to the therapeutic

delay they may cause, be familiar with the following paradigm: *the more*   25
non-indicated tests you order, the more false positive results are obtained,
which in turn compel you to order more tests which lead to additional,
potentially harmful, diagnostic and therapeutic interventions. Eventually,
you loss the controls...

What are the reasons for unnecessary tests? The etiology is a combination of ignorance, lack of confidence, and laziness. When abdominal
emergencies are initially assessed by non-surgeons who do not "understand" the abdomen, unnecessary imaging is requested to compensate
for ignorance. Junior clinicians who lack confidence tend to order tests
"just to be sure – not to miss" a rare disorder. And expericned clinicians
occasionally would ask for an abdominal CT over the phone in order to
procrastinate. Isn't it easier to ask for a CT rather than to drive to the
hospital in the middle of the night and examine the patient: "let's do the
CT and decide in the morning...".

An occasional surgical trainee finds it difficult to understand
"what's wrong with excessive testing?" "Well" we tell him or her, "Why do
we need you at all? Let us all go home instead, and instruct our ER nurses
to drive all patients with abdominal pain through a predetermined line
of tests and imaging modalities". Patients are not cars on a production
line in Detroit. They are individuals who need your continues judgment
and a selective usage of tests.

Be careful before adopting an investigation claimed to be "effective"
by others. You read, for example, that in a Boston ivory tower routine CT
of the abdomen has been proven cost-effective in the diagnosis of acute
appendicitis. Before succumbing to the temptation to order a CT for any
suspected acute appendicitis check out whether the methods used in the
original study can be duplicated in your own environment. Do you have
senior radiologists to read the CT at 3 o'clock at night – or would the CT
be reported on only in the morning-after the appendix is, or should be,
in the formalin jar?

26   Diagnostic Laparoscopy

This is an invasive diagnostic tool to be used in the operating room, after the decision to intervene has been already taken. It has a selective role as discussed in chapter 41.

The more the noise – the less the fact

4 Who Should Look After the "Acute Abdomen" and Where?

Everybody's business is nobody's business

The majority of patients suspected as having an acute abdomen or other abdominal emergency do not require an operation. Nevertheless, it is you – the surgeon who should take, or be granted, the leadership in assessing, excluding or treating this condition, or at least, play a major role in leading the managing team. To emphasize how crucial this issue is, we dedicate to it an entire chapter – although its scope would fit into a paragraph.

Unfortunately, in "real life", surgeons are denied the primary responsibility. Too often we see patients with mesenteric ischemia (chapter 19) rotting away in medical wards, the surgeon being consulted "to evaluate the abdomen", only when the bowel – and, subsequently, the patient – has become dead. A characteristic scenario is a patient with an abdominal surgical emergency, admitted under the care of non-surgeons who undertake a series of unnecessary, potentially harming and expensive diagnostic and therapeutic procedures. Typically, internists, gastroenterologists, infection-disease specialists and radiologists are involved, each prescribing his own wisdom in isolation. When, finally, the surgeon is called in, he finds the condition difficult to diagnose, partially treated or maltreated. Eventually, the indicated operation is performed, but too late and thus carries a higher morbidity and mortality. The etiology of such chaos is not entirely clear. Motives of power, ego and financial considerations (not of the patient) are surely involved.

The team approach to the acutely ill surgical patient should not be discarded. The team, however, should be led and coordinated by a general surgeon. He is the one who knows the abdomen from within and without. He is the one qualified to call- in consultants from other specialties, to order valuable tests, to veto those which are superfluous and wasteful.

28   And, above all, he is the one who will eventually decide that enough is enough and the patient needs to be taken to the operating room.

Continuity of care is a 'sine qua non' in the optimal care of the acute abdomen as the clinical picture, which may change rapidly, is a major determinant in the choice of therapy and its timing. Such patients need to be frequently re-assessed by the same clinician that should be a surgeon. Any deviation from this may be hazardous to the patient; this is our personal experience and that which is repeated 'ad nauseum' in the literature. But why should we be re-inventing the wheel? Why don't we learn? The place for the patient with acute abdominal conditions is on the surgical floor, surgical ICU, or in the OR and under the care of a surgeon – yourself! Do not shade off your responsibilities.

5 Optimizing the Patient

When physiology is disrupted –
attempts at restoring anatomy are futile

The preparation of the patient for surgery may be as crucial
as the operation itself

It's four a.m. and you assess your patient as having an "acute abdomen" – probably due to a perforated viscus. Clearly your patient need an emergency laparotomy; what is left to decide is what efforts, and for how long, should be invested in his optimization before the operation.

Optimization is a double edge sword: spending too much time in trying to "stabilize" an exanguinating patient is an exercise in futility for he will die. Conversely, rushing to surgery with a hypovolemic patient, who suffers from intestinal obstruction, is a recipe for disaster. The issues to be discussed here are:

- Why pre-operative optimization at all?
- What are the goals of optimization?
- Who needs optimization?
- How to do it?

Why Is Pre-operative Optimization Necessary?

Simply, because volume-depleted patients do not tolerate the anesthesia and operation. The induction of general anesthesia and muscle relaxation causes systemic vasodilatation, thus depressing the compensatory – anti-shock physiological mechanisms. On opening the abdomen, intra-peritoneal pressure suddenly declines, allowing pooling of blood in the venous system, which, in turn, depresses cardiac output. An emergency

30   laparotomy in an under resuscitated patient may result in a cardiac arrest even before the operation started. In addition, the intra-operative fluid requirements are unpredictable: do you want to start with a volume-depleted patient, having to chase your tail?

What Are the Goals of Optimization?

Patients awaiting an emergency laparotomy need optimization for two main reasons: *hypovolemia or "sepsis"*. Both conditions cause tissue-under-perfusion and both are treated initially with volume expansion. The chief goal of pre-operative optimization is to improve the delivery of oxygen to the cells. The more severe and prolonged is the cellular hypoxia, the more pronounced will be the resulting cellular dysfunction, SIRS, organ failure and outcome (chapter 38).

In sick surgical patients, unlike the medical ones-optimization means VOLUME and more volume – a lot of fluids. (This is however not true in patients who bleed actively – here optimization means control of the hemorrhage!)

Who Needs Optimization?

Surgical patients often "look" sick. The appearance of the patient usually gives an important first impression; add to it tachycardia, tachypnea, hypotension, mental confusion, and poor peripheral perfusion.

Only basic laboratory studies are necessary: *Hemoconcentration*-reflected in an abnormally high hemoglobin and hematocrit, implies either severe dehydration or extracellular "third space" fluid sequestration. *Urine analysis* with a high specific gravity provides similar information. *Electrolyte imbalance* and associated *prerenal azotemia* again imply volume depletion. *Arterial blood gas* measurement gives critical infor-

mation regarding respiratory function and tissue perfusion. *Note that in*   31
the emergency surgical patient metabolic acidosis almost always means
lactic acidosis – associated with inadequate tissue oxygenation and
anaerobic metabolism at the cellular level. Other causes of metabolic
acidosis, such as renal failure, diabetic ketoacidosis or toxic poisoning are
possible but extremely unlikely. Base excess (BE) is a useful parameter to
look at: a negative base excess of more than minus – 6 is a marker of
significant metabolic acidosis, adverse prognosis and hence the need for
aggressive resuscitation.

All patients with any degree of the above physiological abnormalities
need optimization. Naturally, the magnitude of your efforts should
correlate with the severity of the disturbances.

Measurement of the Severity of Illness

An experience surgeon can "eye-ball" his or her patient and estimate
how "sick they are". But terms such "very sick", "critically ill" or
"moribund" mean different things to different people. We recommend
therefore that you become familiar with a universal physiological
scoring system which measures how really sick is your patient. A scoring
system which was validated in most emergency surgical situations is the
APACHE II (Acute Physiological And Chronic Health Evaluation).
(Figure 5.1). It measures the physiological consequences of acute disease
while taking into consideration the patient's pre-morbid state and age.
The scores are easily measured from readily available basic clinical and
laboratory variables and correlate with the eventual morbidity and
mortality (Figure 5.2). A score of 10 and below represents a relatively
mild disease, a score above 20 signals a critical illness. Instead of telling
your chief resident that this patient is "really sick" you'll say: "his
APACHE II- is 29". Now it is clear to everyone involved that the patient is
moribund.

PHYSIOLOGIC VARIABLE	HIGH ABNORMAL RANGE					LOW ABNORMAL RANGE			
	+4	+3	+2	+1	0	+1	+2	+3	+4
1. Temperature rectal (°C)	≥41°	39°-40.9°		38.5°-38.9°	36°-38.4°	34°-35.9°	32°-33.9°	30°-31.9°	≤29.9°
2. Mean arterial pressure	≥160	130-159	110-129		70-109		50-69		≤49
3. Heart rate (ventricular response)	≥180	140-179	110-139		70-109		55-69	40-54	≤39
4. Respiratory rate (non-ventilated or ventilated)	≥50	35-49		25-34	12-24	10-11	6-9		≤5
5. Oxygenation: A-aDO$_2$ or PaO$_2$ (mmHg) a) FiO$_2$ > 0.5: record A-aDO$_2$	≥500	350-499	200-349		< 200				
b) FiO$_2$ < 0.5: record only PaO$_2$					> 70	61-70		55-60	< 55
6. Arterial pH	≥7.7	7.6-7.69		7.5-7.59	7.33-7.49		7.25-7.32	7.15-7.24	< 7.15
7. Serum Sodium	≥180	160-179	155-159	150-154	130-149		120-129	111-119	≤ 110
8. Serum Potassium	≥7	6-6.9		5.5-5.9	3.5-5.4	3-3.4	2.5-2.9		> 2.5
9. Serum creatinine (mg/dl)	≥3.5	2-3.4	1.5-1.9		0.6-1.4		< 0.6		
10. Hematocrit (%)	≥60		50-59.9	46-49.9	30-45.9		20-29.9		< 20
11. White Blood Count	≥40		20-39.9	15-19.9	3-14.9		1-2.9		< 1
12. Glasgow coma score	15 - GCS =								

Total acute physiology score (APS) = Sum of the 12 individual variable points =

Serum HCO$_3$ (venous-mmol/l) | ≥52 | 41-51.9 | 32-40.9 | | 22-31.9 | | 18-21.9 | 15-17.9 | < 15

A   Total acute physiology score (APS)   (Circle appropriate response)

Glasgow Coma Scale

verbal - nonintubated
Eyes open:
4 - spontaneously   5 - oriented and controverses
3 - to verbal   4 - disoriented and talks
2 - to painful stimuli   3 - inappropriate words
1 - no response   2 - incomprehensible sounds
   1 - no response

Motor response: verbal - intubated
6 - to verbal command   5 - seems able to talk
5 - localizes to pain   3 - questionable ability to talk
4 - with draws to pain   1 - generally unresponsive
3 - decorticate
2 - decerebrate
1 - no response

B   **Age Points**

Age	Points
≤ 44	0
45-54	2
55-64	3
65-74	5
≥ 75	6

Age Points =

C   **Chronic Health Points**

If any of the 5 CHE categories is answered with yes give +5 points for non-operative or emergency postoperative patients.
- Liver   Cirrhosis with PHT or encephalopathy
- Cardiovascular   Class IV angina or at rest or with minimal self-care activities
- Pulmonary   Chronic hypoxemic or hypercapnoe or polycythemic of PHT > 40 mm Hg
- Kidney   Chronic peritoneal or hemodialysis
- Immune   Immune compromised host

Chronic Health Points =

Apache-II Score   (Sum of [A]+[B]+[C])

[A] APS points
\+ [B] Age points
\+ [C] Chronic Health points

=   Total Apache-II

Fig. 5.1. Acute Physiological and Chronic Health Evaluation

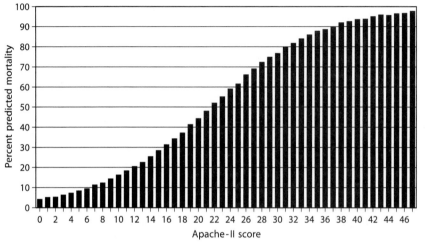

Fig. 5.2. Eventual morbidity and mortality in emergency abdominal surgery

How To Do It?

Despite all that fancy ICU environment, which may or may not be available to you, the optimization of the surgical patient is simple. It can be accomplishable anywhere and requires minimal facilities. All you want is to *better oxygenate the blood and have it better pumped into the tissues.* You do not need a five-star ICU but you do have to stick around with the patient! Writing orders and going to bed (until the operation) will unnecessarily prolong the optimization and delay the operation. So stay with the patient, monitor his progress and be there to decide when enough is enough.

Oxygenation

You know how to oxygenate the patient: any patient who requires
optimization should receive at least oxygen by mask. Look at the patient
and his pulse oxymetry or arterial blood gasses: evidence of hypoventi-
lation or poor oxygenation is an indication for endotracheal intubation
and mechanical ventilation. Do not temporize: the patient will need
intubation anyway so why not now? Remember, pain and distention
associated with the abdominal catastrophe impedes ventilation. Effective
analgesia would impair ventilation further. If nasogastric tube is not
already in situ this is the time to insert one – before intubation: to
decompress the distended stomach and prevent aspiration during the
procedure.

Restoration of Volume

Now after your patient is well oxygenated you must see to it that the
oxygen arrives where it is needed, by restoring blood volume. This is
accomplished by intra-venous infusion of crystalloids such as saline or
Ringer's Lactate. Forget about the much more expensive colloids such as
plasma, albumin or solutions containing synthetic organic macromole-
cules such as Hemastarch or low molecular weight dextran; their
theoretical advantages have never been translated to better results.
Hypertonic saline resuscitation may theoretically be advantageous but is
an investigational therapy at present. Blood and blood products are
given if necessary as discussed below.

   How much crystalloid to infuse? A good rule of thumb is that *the
hypovolemic surgical patient needs more volume than you think he needs
and much more than what the nursing staff thinks he needs.* We assume
that your patient has already a large bore IV catheter in situ – so just
hook it up to the solution and open the valve – let it run! You run in a

liter and hang up another; how much is enough? At this stage you need   35
to assess the *effectiveness of what you do.*

Measurement of Effectiveness of Treatment

The only goal of non-operative treatment in the emergency surgical
patient is the restoration of *adequate tissue perfusion!* This endpoint is
recognized *by physical examination* and measurement of *urinary output,*
in conjunction with the information provided by *selective* invasive
monitoring and laboratory studies.

With fluid resuscitation one hopes to see improvement of tissue
perfusion by normalization of vital signs and improvement in the visible
peripheral circulation. Resolution of hypotension, mental confusion,
tachypnea and tachycardia may be either partially or fully. *Postural
hypotension* reflects a significant deficit in the circulating blood volume.
Remember that the usual response to a change in position from supine
to upright is an increase in the systolic blood pressure – a widening of the
pulse pressure. Consequently, when a narrowing of the pulse pressure is
seen when the patient sits up then postural hypotension is present. With
fluid resuscitation mottling of the skin and the palpable temperature of
the fingers and toes may improve. *Capillary refill* is a clinical test, which
observes the peripheral circulation in the nail bed. The nail bed blanches
when pressed and should return to its normal pink color in less than
two seconds. Fluid resuscitation aims to correct this subtle abnormality
of the peripheral circulation as well.

Urine Output

A Foley urinary bladder catheter is a sine qua non – in any patient requiring optimization. It allows an accurate, if indirect, measurement of tissue

36   perfusion and *adequacy of fluid resuscitation* as reflected in the urine
output. Your aim is at least one half to one milliliter of urine per
kilogram of the patient's weight in each hour. This is the single best sign
of adequate tissue perfusion associated with successful fluid resuscitation.

Invasive Monitoring

You are of course are familiar with the central venous and the Swan-
Ganz -pulmonary arterial catheters. These are tools which permit
"special studies" to be carried out rapidly and on an ongoing basis. The
downside of such devices is that they are invasive, expensive, often
inaccurate, and associated with potential life-threatening complications.
Invasive hemodynamic monitoring provides endpoint measurements
which, in conjunction with urinary output, indicate the adequacy of fluid
resuscitation.

The *central venous catheter* measures central venous pressure
(CVP) which is a product of the venous return (i.e. blood volume) and
right ventricular function. *Low CVP always means hypovolemia but a
high CVP can signify either over-expansion of blood volume or cardiac
failure.* So aim for an adequate urinary output with a CVP in the normal
range – around 12 cm' H_2O. When the CVP rises above the normal range
and the urinary output is still not adequate then either the cardiac
function is impaired or the measurement is in error. False elevations in
CVP are caused by abnormally high intra-thoracic or intra-abdominal
pressure, which is directly transmitted to the great thoracic veins. The
message is clear: *as long as the urine output is not adequate and the CVP
is low – pour in the fluids.* But remember: your patient may be far behind
on fluid in the presence of a high or normal CVP. And another hint:
the absolute CVP reading means less than its trend; it is when a low or
normal CVP suddenly jumps up you have to slow the fluids.

The Swan-Ganz

The Swan-Ganz measures pulmonary capillary wedge pressure, which reflects the volume status and left cardiac function. Like the CVP catheter, the "Swan" is used in conjunction with the urinary output. We aim for a normal "wedge" pressure (around 14 mmHg) in conjunction with an adequate urinary output. As with the CVP – a low "wedge" always means hypovolemia, a high "wedge" on the other hand, may indicate either a volume overload, or dysfunction of the left heart. With the Swan-Ganz in situ you can calculate and derive information about cardiac function (cardiac output and cardiac index), adrenergic response to injury or illness (peripheral vascular resistance) or tissue perfusion (oxygen consumption and oxygen delivery). A normal cardiac index is a good confirmatory endpoint for resuscitation and, if pre-existing renal failure is present, is a good independent endpoint. When the wedge pressure is normal or high and the urinary output and cardiac index are still low then pharmacological intervention with inotropic agents may be indicated.

We know that intensivists and junior doctors like to insert central lines and especially Swan -Ganz catheters. Being invasive and able to measure sophisticated data is "fun" and clinically attractive. But invasive monitoring is far from being a panacea. Wedge pressures are notoriously inaccurate in emergency surgical patients – prone to false high reading similarly to the CVP. The Swan-Ganz catheters are expensive, predisposed to complications and above all – they very rarely add something to the management of your patients. Did you know that no good studies exist to support its use? And consider this: when was it the last time when your anesthetist *really* effectively used, during the operation, the Swan Ganz you placed pre-operatively? We can not remember such a case.

38   Laboratory

The information provided by laboratory studies is easy to interpret. Aim for resolution of hemoconcentration, normalization of electrolyte, BUN and creatinine levels and resolution of metabolic acidosis. As mentioned previously – look at the BE, if persistently negative- the oxygen depth at the tissue levels has not resolved.

Blood and Blood Products

Blood products such whole blood, packed red blood cells, fresh frozen plasma, cryoprecipitate or platelet concentrate, are indicated selectively to restore oxygen carrying capacity in actively bleeding or chronically anemic patients and to correct clotting abnormalities if present. Do not forget however the blood bank blood is a double edge sword. Beyond the "usual" and well-known complications of transfusion, blood is immuno-suppressive – increasing the probability of post postoperative infections. In addition, the more blood you give the higher is the risk of postoperative organ system dysfunction.

Do not forget that re-hydration with crystalloids may unmask chronic anemia as the hematocrit falls with volume expansion.

Suggested Steps In Volume Optimization

- Institute intravenous fluid therapy and if signs of intestinal dysfunction such as nausea, vomiting or abdominal distension are present then designate nil per mouth (NPO) and, in more severe cases, nasogastric suction. Intravenous crystalloid may be started at a basic rate of 100 to 200 ml per hour with the addition of

boluses of 250 to 500 ml given over intervals of 15 to 30 minutes.
We advice, however, to sit by your patient and completely open the
valve of the transfusion set, despite the nurses desire to keep it on
a pump.

- Institute procedures for monitoring the effectiveness of treatment
  including serial physical exam, Foley catheter placement and, in
  more severe cases, central venous catheter placement. Swan Ganz?
  Please, be selective with this "gimmick".
- If the main underlying problem is hemorrhage, institute transfusion
  of packed red blood cells-typed and cross matched if there is time,
  type specific only if there is not.
- Titrate the rate of fluid administration in light of the results of
  monitoring. Increase or decrease the basic rate of fluid flow and
  give additional bolus infusions as necessary.
- *After* the restoration of intravascular fluid volume address any
  residual signs of physiologic dysfunction with inotropic agents to
  improve cardiac output and, possibly, an afterload reducing agent
  to improve myocardial oxygen supply and ease the workload of the
  heart. There is no shame in looking up the dosage and administration recommendations while the fluid is going in.
- Wheel the patient directly to the operating room yourself. Do not
  wait for the porter – isn't he always late?
- If the basic problem is ongoing hemorrhage then forget this list
  and go directly to the operating room. The best resuscitation in
  actively bleeding patients is the surgical control of the source.
  In addition, *pre-operative over resuscitation and transfusion may in
  fact increase the blood loss.*

40   When Enough Is Enough?

The above steps in optimization are done with the aim of correcting physiologic derangements as much as possible but without unnecessarily delaying operative intervention. There is no magic formula for achieving this balance. The disease process itself will determine the duration of pre-operative optimization. At one end of the spectrum uncontrolled hemorrhage will require immediate operative intervention after only partial fluid resuscitation or none at all. At the other end of the spectrum intestinal obstruction that has been developing over several days will require a more complete resuscitation prior to operation. As in life in general, most cases will fall somewhere in between-which means around 3 hours. Stubborn attempts to "improve" a "non-responder" beyond 6 hours are counter-productive.

Conclusions

The key to pre-operative optimization in emergency surgery is oxygenation of the blood and intravenous fluid resuscitation with crystalloid solutions. The only goal of resuscitation is the restoration of adequate tissue perfusion to supply oxygen to the suffocating mitochondria. Accomplish it aggressively to reduce intra- and postoperative complications.

> **These old folks maintain a fragile system quite well...**
> **until it gets disturbed-like a card house**

6   Pre-operative Antibiotics

Most men die of their remedies, not of their diseases (Molière)

It is common practice to administer broad-spectrum antibiotics before a laparotomy for an acute surgical condition or trauma. In this situation, antibiotics are either *therapeutic* or *prophylactic*. Therapeutic antibiotics are given for an already established, tissue invasive, infection (e.g. perforated appendicitis). Prophylaxis involves the administration of these agents in the absence of infection, with the objective of reducing the anticipated incidence of infections which result from existing (e.g. penetrating injury of the colon) or potential (e.g. gastrotomy to suture a bleeding ulcer) contamination during the operative procedure. It is very important to distinguish between *contamination* and *infection* (chapter 10) as only the latter requires postoperative antibiotic administration, a topic to be discussed in the postoperative section (chapter 32). *Therapeutic* antibiotics assist the surgeon and the natural peritoneal defenses to eradicate an established infection. *Prophylactic* antibiotics prevent postoperative infections of the laparotomy wound; they are neither meant to prevent pulmonary or urinary infections nor the occurrence of intra-abdominal abscesses. *Even dummies know that antibiotics are only an adjunct to the proper surgical management of contamination and infection* (chapter 10).

When Should You Start Antibiotics?

If intra-abdominal contamination or infection is evident or strongly suspected pre-operatively, administer antibiotics immediately – "the sooner the better". In case of delay to proceed with the laparotomy, give a second dose of pre-incisional antibiotics in the operating room. Pre-incisional administration is best in cases where contamination is expected to occur intra-operatively. Some surgeons, however, prefer to

42 await the operative findings before giving antibiotics. Should, for example, the acute appendicitis prove as "simple-phlegmonous" (chapter 22), or the blunt trauma not breaching the lumen of a hollow viscus (chapter 27), they would avoid antibiotics altogether. Alternatively, if contamination or infection is encountered, antibiotics are started a few minutes after abdominal entry, with no apparent disadvantage. Another issue has been the possibility that antibiotics liberate endotoxin from the killed bacteria; this led some surgeons to believe that evacuation of pus (containing the source of endotoxin) should be a prerequisite to commencing antimicrobial therapy.

Our position is to administer a dose of antibiotics *prior to all* emergency abdominal operations. When infection or contamination is present, or when contamination is expected to occur, the prophylactic or therapeutic value of antibiotics is obvious. In view of the beneficial effects of prophylactic antibiotics in certain elective, clean procedures we assume that the same may be true in the acutely ill patient who is subjected to laparotomy, even in the absence of contamination or infection. The clinical significance of the antibiotic-generated endotoxemia is presently unknown.

Not uncommonly, we observe surgeons who in the "peri-operative chaos" forget to administer antibiotics. To compensate for their failure, they order antibiotics after the operation. This is utterly futile! Are dirty hands washed before or after the meal? The fate of the operative wound is sealed by intra-operative events, including timely administration of antibiotics. Nothing done *after* the operation can change the outcome of the wound (chapter 40).

What Agents to Administer?

Contrary to what is preached by drug companies and their various beneficiaries or representatives, the choice of drugs is straightforward. Many

single drug or combination-regimens are available and equally effective;   43
the most recent and expensive not necessarily being better. The bacterial
flora of abdominal contamination or infection derives from the gastrointestinal tract and is predictable. When a drop of feces leaks into the
peritoneal cavity, it contains more than 400 different species of bacteria;
only a handful of these are involved in the ensuing infection. Thus, from
the initial plethora of contaminating bacteria, the inoculum is spontaneously reduced and *simplified* to include only a few organisms that
survive outside their natural environment. These are the endotoxin-
generating facultative anaerobes such as *E.coli* and obligate anaerobes,
such as *Bacteroides fragilis*; which act in synergy. Any agent or combination of agents that effectively kills these target bacteria can be used.

The once popular "triple regimen" of the 1970 s (ampicillin, an
aminoglycoside, and metronidazole or clindamycin) has become obsolete.
Enterococcus, frequently isolated in experimental and clinical peritonitis,
is clinically almost non-significant as a pathogen in the peritoneal cavity
and does not require to be "covered" with ampicillin. Aminoglycosides
are markedly more nephrotoxic (especially in critically ill patients), are
inefficient in the low pH of the infected peritoneal environment, and are
no longer the first choice of antibiotics in the initial treatment of intra-
abdominal infection. Surgeons tend to be creatures of habit, desperately
clinging to dogmas passed on by their mentors; the "triple regimen" is
one such dogma that risks to be carried into the 21 century through
ignorance. There are numerous agents on the market you can chose
from. You may use whichever agent, as a 'monotherapy' or in combination – as along as *E.coli* and *B.fragilis* are "covered".

In abdominal emergencies, the same agent should be used for prophylaxis and treatment. An initial dose of the appropriate drug is given
pre-operatively and, if indicated by the intra-operative findings, can be
continued following the operation. The common (mal)practice of starting
with a "weak" agent (e.g. cephazolin) before the operation and converting
to the "strong" regimen is baseless.

44   In the course of the fluid-resuscitation of hypovolemic patients, antimicrobials may be "diluted", reducing the availability of antimicrobial drugs at sites of contamination or infection. In these cases, especially in the trauma patient, higher initial doses should be used: *"sooner and more is better than less and longer"*.

In conclusion: start antibiotics prior to any emergency laparotomy; whether to continue administration after the operation depends on your findings. Know the target flora and use the cheapest and simplest regimen. The bacteria cannot be confused, nor should you be!

7   Family, Ethics, Informed Consent and Medicolegal Considerations

Doctor, my doctor, what do you say...?
(Philip Roth)

The wind whistles through the cracks in your call room window when the ER calls and suddenly you find yourself in the maelstrom of that environment, speaking to a small group of extremely anxious strangers – having to explain that an immediate operation will be required to save their beloved one. The OR is ready.

Providing informed consent is a practical combination of salesmanship, ethical problem solving and psychological nurturing. It involves the rapid marketing of one's own skills and plan for treatment. It requires the recruitment of the patient and their family as allies in the decision making process. Rather than a legal requirement, however, informed consent requires an ethical commitment to one's patient, one's peers and to one's self.

Salesmanship

Begin by explaining your proposed treatment using the same words and language, which you might use in speaking to one of your non-physician parents. Describe the expected benefits of operation and what the consequences of alternative treatment approaches might be. Offer several scenarios; take a case of obstructing carcinoma of the sigmoid colon for example. At one end of the spectrum is nonoperative management, which almost certainly will result in a slow and difficult death. At the other end of the spectrum is rapid recovery from operation with long term "cure" of the disease. In between lie the potential difficulties of peri-operative complication or death, recovery with disability or recurrent

46   disease. It is crucial that you believe in the plan of treatment, which you propose. If this is not the case, and the plan is not acceptable to you, but dictated to you from above – let the responsible person to conduct his own "negotiations".

"Sell" yourself to the patient and family as a scientific expert who recognizes the needs of another person and is participating with them in solving a difficult problem. Include a description, with approximate probabilities, of the most common "problems" (complications) for the proposed procedure in your particular patient. You will need to make an estimate based on general and specific information. For example, the risk of mortality for elective colon resection may be negligible but in an elderly patient with acute colonic obstruction and hypoalbuminemia the odds of dying may be one in four (chapter 5). Discuss "general" potential postoperative complications such as infection, hemorrhage (and risk of transfusion), poor healing and death. Then mention the unique complications specific to the procedure you are proposing to undertake, such as common bile duct injury in laparoscopic cholecystectomy.

It is crucial that before any major emergency abdominal operation you emphasize that a re-operation may be necessary – based on your operative finding or if a problem subsequently develops. This would drastically facilitate the "negotiation" with the family when a re-operation is indeed indicated (chapter 37); they would understand that the re-operation represents a "continued management effort" rather than a "complication". Minor complications, such as phlebitis arising from peri-operative IV therapy, may contribute to information overload and probably should be omitted. Try to conduct the above "script" in a relatively quiet setting-away from the usual chaos of the ER, SICU or the OR. Use simple language and repeat yourself ad libidum: stressed members of family have difficulty to grasp what you say. Offer the opportunity to ask questions, continuously assess whether they understand what you say; the more they do now, the less "problems" you'll have with them if complications subsequently develop. Be "human", friendly, emphatic but professional. A good trick is to remind yourself from time to time that the family you talk to could be yours.

When discussing the prospects of an operation with a patient or a family we find that illustrating the problem and the planned procedure on a blank piece of paper greatly enhances the communication. Your draw schematically the obstructed colon: "here is the colon, this is the obstructing lesion and here is the segment we want to remove; we hope to be able to join this piece of bowel to that one, a colostomy may however be needed, this is the place it will be brought out...". Below the drawing you write the diagnosis and the name of the planned operation. At the end of the consultation you'll be surprised to see how carefully members of the family re-study the piece of paper you left with them, explaining to each other the diagnosis and operation.

The Family

The patient's family is your greatest ally in promoting your plan of action. By involving them at an early point in the decision-making process you may be able to make them partners in the relationship which you share with the patient. By avoiding the family you may alienate potential allies or worsen an already "difficult" group. The "difficult family" is common. Long submerged conflicts and feelings of guilt tend to surface when a member of the group becomes ill. Recruit them as allies by offering them a chance to participate, by "reading" the nuances of their relationships and by confidently and continuously selling yourself as a knowledgeable and compassionate advisor. Use your first meeting with the family to make a good impression and gain their trust so that you will continue to be trusted when a complication arises or when further therapy becomes necessary.

48   Ethical Problem Solving

In order to sell a particular product or idea one must believe in it. In other words-based on your knowledge and experience the operation you offer should appear ethical to you. It is ethical if it is expected to either:

*   save the patient's life,
*   prolong his life,
*   palliate his symptoms,
*   achieve these with a reasonable benefit/risk ratio.

At the same time you must be also convinced that there are no non-operative treatment modalities which are safer and/or as effective as your proposed operation. The burden of proof is on you!

Medicolegal Considerations

The medicolegal dangers associated with emergency abdominal surgery greatly depend on where you practice. In some countries surgeons can "get away" with almost anything, in other countries – emergency surgery is a legal minefield. There are a few simple but well proven tactics to prevent lawsuits against you:

*   Have the patient and family "on your side" (as mentioned above) by being emphatic, caring, honest, open, informative, and at the same time professional. Young surgeons tend to be over-optimistic – trying to "cheer-up" the family. Often they would come out of the operating room, assuming a 'tired hero' pose – to announce: "It was smooth and easy, I removed the cancer from the colon – relieving the obstruction; I joined then the bowel together-avoiding a colostomy. Yes, your father is stable, he took the operation very well, let's hope he'll be home next week for Easter". Such script is obviously

wrong – raising high hopes and expectations and, consequently – anger and resentment if complications would develop. The "correct" script would be: "the operation was difficult, but we managed to achieve our goals, the cancer is out and we avoided a colostomy. Yes, considering his age and other illnesses he took it well. Let us hope for the best but you must understand that the road to recovery is long and there are still many potential complications to avoid, as I mentioned to you before the operation..."

- Detailed informed consent.
- Documentation. This is crucial as what has not been documented in writing 'did not actually take place'. Your notes can be brief but must encompass the essentials. Prior to an emergency laparotomy for colonic obstruction we would write: "78 YO male patient with hypertension, diabetes and COPD at the background. Three days of abdominal pain plus distention. Abdominal X ray-suggesting a distal large bowel obstruction – confirmed on gastrografin study. APACHE II score on admission 17 – making him a high risk. Therapeutic options, risks and potential complications explained to the patient and family who agreed for an emergency laparotomy. They understand that a colostomy may be needed and that further operations may be necessary." A few years later-in court – this short note will prove invaluable to you!

Avoid Selling AUA's

We compared you above to an astute salesman, interacting with the patient and his family. In this capacity, you, a respected clinician, can easily sell anything to the trusting clients. Be honest with yourself and consider as objectively as possible the risk-benefit ratio of the procedure you are trying to 'sell". How easy it is to convince a worried family that a (futile) operation is indeed necessary for their beloved one. And at the

50   inevitable M & M meeting (chapter 42) you'll explain that the family
       forced the AUA (autopsy under anesthesia) on you...

       **One should only advice surgery if there is a reasonable chance
       of success. To operate without having a chance means to prostitute
       the beautiful art and science of surgery
       (Theodor Billroth)**

Section B:

The Operation

8   The Incision

Incisions heal from side to side, not from end to end,
but length does matter.

When entering the abdomen,
your finger is the best and safest instrument.

The patient now lies on the table, anesthetized and ready for your knife. Before you scrub, carefully examine the relaxed abdomen. Now, you can feel things, which were impossible to feel in the tense and tender belly. You may feel a distended gallbladder in a patient diagnosed as an acute appendicitis, or an appendiceal mass in a patient booked for a cholecystectomy. Yes, this may also occur in days of ultrasound and CT. As a pilot prior the flight, go over the list: antibiotics given? Subcut heparin injected? Is the patient correctly positioned? Now you can go and scrub! You are the Captain of the ship – behave as one: the scene of a surgeon who directly enters the room with his scrubbed hands high in the air is pitiful.

Traditionally, abdominal entry in an emergency situation or for exploratory purposes has been through a generous and easily extensible vertical incision, especially the midline one. Generally speaking, the trans linea alba midline incision is swiftly effected and relatively bloodless. On the other hand, transverse or paramedian vertical incisions are a little more time and blood consuming but are associated with a lower incidence of wound dehiscence and incisional hernia formation. In addition, transverse incisions are known to be "easier" on the patient and his lung function in the postoperative period.

Keeping this in mind, we should be *pragmatic rather than dogmatic* and tailor the incision to the individual patient and his/her disease process. We should take into consideration the urgency of the situation, the site and nature of the condition, the confidence in (or uncertainty about) the preoperative diagnosis, and the build of the patient.

54   *Common sense dictates that the most direct access to the specific intra-abdominal pathology is preferable.* Thus, the biliary system is best approached through a transverse, right subcostal incision. Transverse incisions are easily extensible across, to offer additional exposure; a right subcostal incision can be extended into the left side (as a 'chevron') – offering an excellent view of the entire abdomen. When a normal appendix is uncovered through a limited incision like a McBurney's, one can extend across the midline to deal with any intestinal or pelvic condition. Alternatively, when an upper abdominal process is found, it is perfectly reasonable to close the small right iliac fossa incision and place a new, more appropriate, one.

When the presumptive diagnosis is focused on one or the other side of the abdomen, a paramedian incision offers a more direct access to the troubled spot. The midline incision – bloodless, rapid, and easily extensible – affords superior exposure and versatility; it remains the classic "incision of indecision" – when the site of the abdominal catastrophe is unknown, and the safest approach in trauma.

This is an occasion to mention that a laparotomy without a diagnosis is not a sin! Do not surrender to the prevailing dogma that without a ticket from the CT scanner the patient cannot enter the operating theater. A clinical acute abdomen remains an indication for laparotomy and on many occasions the abdominal wall is the only structure separating the surgeon from the accurate diagnosis.

At what level must the midline incision start and how long should it be? The macho surgeons of the previous generations often screamed: "Do it long. It heals from side to side, not from end to end". Today, in an era of minimally invasive surgery, we are familiar with the advantages of shorter incisions. In the absence of an obvious urgency, enter the abdomen through a short incision and then extend as necessary; but never compromise for a less than adequate exposure or keyhole surgery. Begin with an upper or lower midline incision, directed by your clinically guided assessment; when in doubt start in the midline's center and "sniff" around from there, then extend towards the pathology.

Should You Extend Your Incision into the Thorax?

Very rarely! In the vast majority of cases, the infra-diaphragmatic pathology is approachable through abdominal incisions. The combination of a subcostal and upper midline incision offers an excellent exposure for almost all emergency hepatic procedures, with the exception of retrohepatic venous injuries where insertion of a trans-atrial vena cava shunt necessitates a median sternotomy – usually a futile exercise, anyway. Thoracoabdominal incisions are thus mainly reserved for combined thoracoabdominal trauma.

Knife or Diathermy?

A few studies suggest that the latter is a few minutes slower while the former sheds a few more drops of blood; otherwise results are comparable. We use either. In extreme urgency, gain an immediate entry with a few swift strokes of the knife; otherwise, the diathermy is convenient, especially when performing transverse muscle-cutting incisions. Adequate hemostasis is a crucial surgical principle but do not go overboard chasing the individual erythrocytes and do not reduce to "charcoal" the subcutaneous fat or skin. Subcutaneous hemostatic ligatures behave as a foreign body and are almost never necessary. In fact, most incisional oozers stop spontaneously, after a few minutes, under the pressure of a moist lap pad. It is also unnecessary to "clean" the fascia by sweeping the fat laterally; the more you dissect and "burn", the more inflammation and infection – generating dead tissue – you create!

Keep in Mind Special Circumstances.

If a stoma is anticipated then place the incision away from its planned location. Abdominal re-entry into the "hostile abdomen" of a previously operated patient can be problematic; you may spend more time, sweat

56   and blood, but the real danger is creating inadvertent enterotomies in intestine adherent to the previous incisional scar. This is a common cause of postoperative external bowel fistula! (Chapter 39) The prevailing opinion is to use the previous incision for re-entry, *if possible*. When doing so, however, start a few centimeters below or above the old incision and gain entry into the abdomen through virgin territory. Insert then your finger into the peritoneal cavity and navigate your way safely in, taking down adhesions to abdominal wall, which hamper the insertion of a self–retaining retractor. Essentially, you finished "getting in" when you are able to place a self–retaining retractor to open the belly wide. In a dire emergency or when you expect the abdomen to be exceptionally scarred, it may be prudent to stay away from trouble and create an entirely fresh incision.

Pitfalls

- When in haste, do not forget that the *liver* lies in the upper extreme of the long midline incision, and the *urinary bladder* at its lowermost. Be careful not to damage either.
- When approaching the upper abdomen divide and ligate the *round* hepatic ligament. Leave it long: it could be used to elevate and retract on the liver. Take the opportunity to divide the bloodless *falciform* ligament, which runs from the anterior abdominal wall and the diaphragm to the liver. If left intact it may "tear" off the liver causing irritating bleeding.
- When performing any transverse incision across the midline, do not forget to ligate or transfix the epigastric vessels just behind the rectus abdominis muscles. They may retract and cause a delayed abdominal wall hematoma.

Pray before surgery, but remember God will not alter a faulty incision (Arthur H. Keeney)

9 Abdominal Exploration: Finding What Is Wrong

Never let the skin stand between you and the diagnosis

Not uncommonly, when opening the abdomen, the surgeon knows what to expect inside; the clinical picture and/or ancillary tests direct him onto the disease process (e.g. an acute appendicitis or obstructing sigmoid lesion). On many instances, however, he dips into the unknown, being warned only by the signs of peritoneal irritation, and assuming that the peritoneal cavity is flooded by blood or pus. Usually, the surgeon speculates about the predicted diagnosis but always remains ready for the unexpected. This is what makes emergency abdominal surgery so exciting and demanding: the ever looming surprises and the anxiety about whether you are able, or not, to tackle it competently.

Abdominal Exploration

While the specific sequence and extent of abdominal exploration are to be tailored to the clinical circumstances, the two principal stages of any exploration are:

- The identification of the specific pathology which prompted the laparotomy
- The routine exploration of the peritoneal cavity

Essentially, there is a sharp distinction between a laparotomy for non-traumatic conditions such as bowel obstruction, inflammation or peritonitis, and laparotomy for trauma with intra-abdominal hemorrhage, the later being rarely due to non-traumatic intra-abdominal causes.

So you incise the peritoneum; and what now? Your action depends on the urgency of situation (condition of the patient), mechanisms of abdominal

58   pathology (spontaneous versus trauma), and the initial findings (blood, contamination or pus). Whatever you find, follow the main *priorities*:

- Identify and arrest active bleeding
- Identify and check ongoing contamination

At the same time: *do not be distracted by trivia.* Sarcastically speaking, do not chase isolated red blood cells or bacteria in a patient who is bleeding to death. In other words: do not repair minor mesenteric tears in a patient who is busy exanguinating from a torn inferior vena cava. This is not a joke-surgeons are easily distracted.

Intra-peritoneal Blood

The patient may have suffered a blunt or penetrating injury or no injury at all. You may have been expecting the presence of free intra-peritoneal blood from the findings of hypovolemic shock, peritoneal lavage, or the CT scan. Your action depends on the magnitude of hemorrhage and the degree of resulting hemodynamic compromise. When the abdomen is full of blood, and the patient unstable, you should act swiftly:

Control the Situation:
- Enlarge your initial incision generously
- Eviscerate the bowel completely
- Suck out blood as fast as possible (always have 2 large suckers ready)
- Pack the four quadrants with laparotomy pads tightly

Evacuation of massive hemoperitoneum temporarily aggravates hypovolemia. It releases the tamponade-effect and relieves the intra-abdominal hypertension (chapter 28), resulting in sudden pooling of blood in the venous circulation. At this stage, compress the aorta at its diaphragmatic hiatus and let the anesthetist catch up with fluid and blood requirements. Be patient, do not rush forward; with your fist on the aorta, the abdomen tightly packed, and the patient's vital organs perfusion improving, you have almost all the time in the world. Do not be tempted to continue with the operation, which can result in a successful hemostasis in a dead patient. Relax and plan the next move, remembering that from now on you can afford loosing only a limited amount of blood before the vicious circle of hypothermia, acidosis, and coagulopathy will further frustrate efforts to achieve hemostasis.

Primary Survey

Now you are ready to identify and treat the life-threatening injuries. The initial direction of your search will be guided by the causative mechanisms. In penetrating injury the bleeding source should be at or the vicinity of the missile or knife tract; in blunt trauma, bleeding will probably originate from a ruptured solid organ – the liver, spleen or the pelvic retroperitoneum.

Unpack, suck and re-pack each quadrant consecutively noting where is the blood re-accumulation (active bleeding) or hematoma. Having accurately identified the source (or sources) of bleeding, start definitive hemostasis, the rest of the abdomen being packed away. Simultaneously, if situation permits, control sources of contamination from injured bowel using clamps, staplers or tapes, or re-packing in desperate situations.

Secondary Survey

Now the exanguinating lesion is permanently or temporarily controlled and the patient's hemodynamics stabilized. With less adrenaline floating around you can divert your attention to all the rest, and look more precisely around. With growing experience your abdominal exploration will become more efficient but never less thorough as "missed" abdominal injuries continue to be a common source of preventable morbidity. The practicalities of systematic abdominal exploration are described below.

Intra-peritoneal Contamination or Infection

First you register the offensive fecal smell that denotes abundance of anaerobic bacteria and usually an infective source in the bowel. Equally is true with the finding of fecal – appearing fluid. Note, however, that neglected infections from any cause can be pseuofeculant due to the predominance of anaerobes. When on opening the peritoneum air escapes with a hiss, be aware that a viscus has perforated. In the non- trauma situation this usually implies perforated peptic ulcer or sigmoid diverticulitis. Bile-staining of the exudate point to pathology in the biliary tract, gastroduodenum or proximal small bowel. Dark stout – beer fluid and fat necrosis hints to pancreatic necrosis or its infection – in the lesser sac. *Whatever the nature of contamination or pus, suck and mop it away as soon as possible.*

Generally, bile directs you proximally and feces distally; but "simple" pus can derive from anywhere. When its source remains elusive start a systematic search keeping in mind all potential intra and retroperitoneal sources "from the esophagus to the rectum". Be persistent with your search; we recall a case of spontaneous perforation of the rectum in a young male; twice explored by experienced surgeons who failed to appreciate the minute hole deep at the Douglas pouch. It was found during the third operation.

Occasionally, however, the root of contamination or secondary peritonitis is not found. A Gram-stain, disclosing a solitary bacteria-as

opposed to a few – would support the diagnosis of *primary peritonitis,*   61
since secondary peritonitis (i.e. secondary to a visceral pathology) is
always poymicrobial. More about this in the next chapter (chapter 10).

The Direction and Practicalities of Exploration

This depends on the reason for the laparotomy; here we bring a general
plan.

The peritoneal cavity is comprised of *two compartments*: the *supra-mesocolic* and the *infra-mesocolic compartment.* The dividing line is the
transverse (meso)colon which in a xipho-pubic midline incision is located
approximately in the center of the incision. It is important to develop
and adhere to a fixed routine of abdominal exploration, which will include
both compartments. Our preference is to begin with the infra-mesocolic
compartment: the transverse colon is retracted upwards and the small
bowel is eviscerated, and the recto-sigmoid is identified. Exploration begins with the pelvic reproductive organs in the female, and then attention
is turned to a systematic inspection and palpation of the rectosigmoid,
progressing in a retrograde fashion to the left, transverse and then right
colon and cecum, including inspection of the mesocolon. The assistant
follows the exploration with successive movements of a hand-held
retractor to retract the edge of the surgical incision and enable good
visualization of the abdominal structure, which is the focus of attention.
Exploration then proceeds in a retrograde fashion from the ileo-cecal
valve to the ligament of Triez, with special care being taken to inspect
both "anterior" and "posterior" aspects of each loop of bowel as well as
it's mesentery. This concludes the exploration of the infra-mesocolic
compartment.

Attention is then turned to the *supra-mesocolic compartment.* The
transverse colon is pulled down, and the surgeon inspects and palpates

62

the liver, gallbladder, stomach (including the proper placement of a nasogastric tube), and spleen. Special care should be taken to avoid iatrogenic damage to the spleen caused by pulling hard on the body of the stomach or the greater omentum. A complete abdominal exploration also includes entry into the lesser peritoneal sac, which is best undertaken through the gastrocolic omentum. This omentum is usually only a thin avascular membrane on the left side, and this should therefore be the preferred entry site into the lesser sac. Special care should be taken to avoid injury to the transverse mesocolon which may be adherent to the gastrocolic omentum, and thus misdirect the surgeon who is convinced that he is entering the sac when in fact he or she is cutting a hole in the mesentery. The gastrocolic omentum is divided between ligatures bringing the body and tail of the pancreas into full view.

The key to the exploration of retroperitoneal structures include two mobilization maneuvers which should be employed whenever access to the retroperitoneum is deemed necessary:

- *"Kocher's maneuver"* is mobilization of the duodenal loop and the head of the pancreas by incising the thin peritoneal membrane (posterior peritoneum) overlying the lateral aspect of the duodenum and gradually lifting the duodenum and pancreatic head medially. This maneuver is also the key to surgical exposure of the right kidney and the right adrenal gland. Kocher's maneuver may be extended further caudad along the "white line" on the lateral aspect of the right colon all the way down to the cecum. This extension allows medial rotation of the right colon and affords good exposure of the right-sided retroperitoneal structures such as the inferior vena cava, iliac vessels and the right ureter. Further extension of this incision angles around the caecum and continues in a supero-medial direction along the line of fusion of the small bowel mesentery to the posterior abdominal wall. Thus it is possible to mobilize and reflect the small bowel upwards, the so-called *Catell-Braasch*

maneuver. This affords optimal exposure of the entire infra-   63
mesocolic retroperitoneum, including the aorta and it's infra-renal
branches.

- The second key mobilization maneuver is called "*left sided Kocher*"
  or "*medial visceral rotation*" and is used especially to gain access
  to the entire length of the abdominal aorta and to the left-sided
  retroperitoneal viscera. Depending on the structure to be exposed
  this maneuver begins either lateral to the spleen (spleno-phrenic
  and spleno-renal ligament) working caudaly or in the "white line"
  of Toldt lateral to the junction of the descending and sigmoid
  colon, working cephalad. The peritoneum is incised and the viscera
  are gradually mobilized medially, including the left colon, spleen
  and tail of pancreas. The right kidney can either be mobilized or
  left in situ, depending on the surgical target of the exploration.

In cases of *spontaneous hemoperitoneum* you'll have to look for a ruptured
aortic, iliac or visceral arterial aneurysm, ectopic pregnancy, bleeding
hepatic tumors or spontaneous rupture of an enlarge spleen. In penetrating trauma you'll follow the entry-exit tract, taking in consideration
the missile's energy, velocity and potential to fragmentize. *Wherever
there is an entry wound in a viscus or blood vessel look for the exit one!*
The latter may lie concealed on the lesser sac wall of the stomach, the
retroperitoneal surface of the duodenum, or the mesenteric edge of the
small bowel. It is the blunt abdominal injury, however, which requires
the most extensive and less directed search; from the surface of both
hemi-diaphragms to the pelvis, from gutter to gutter, all solid organs, the
whole length of the GI tract, and the retroperitoneum. (the retroperitoneum selectively, as discussed in chapter 27). The exact sequence of
exploration is of lesser importance than its exactness.

64 Additional Points: Grading the Severity of Injury

Abdominal exploration for trauma ends with a strategic decision about the subsequent steps. Forget at this stage the many available injury organ scales, which have an academic value; from the operating surgeon's point of view there are essentially two patterns of visceral damage: "minor trouble" and "major trouble".

- "*Minor trouble*" are easily fixable injuries, either because the injured organ is accessible or the surgical solution is straightforward (e.g. splenectomy, suture of mesenteric bleeders, or a colon perforation). There is no immediate danger of exanguination or loss of surgical control. Under these circumstances you can immediately proceed with definitive repair.

- "*Major trouble*" is when the spontaneous condition or injury is not easily controlled or immediately fixable because of complexity or inaccessibility (e.g. a high-grade liver injury, a major retroperitoneal vascular injury in the supra-mesocolic compartment or destruction of the pancreatoduodenal complex). Here the secret of success is to STOP the operation when temporary (usually digital or manual) control of bleeding is achieved. Take time to optimize the surgical attack on the injured organ. Update all members of the operating team on the operative plan. Instruct your anesthesiologist to use the time to hemodynamically stabilize the patient and to get more blood products (often you have to think for your anesthetist-don't assume that he is awake). Order an autotransfusion device and a full range of vascular and thoracotomy instruments to be brought in. This is also the appropriate time to seek more competent help, and to plan the operative attack, including additional exposure and mobilization. Such preparations are crucial for the survival of your patient.

Remember: very often the initial exploration of the abdomen in the trauma   65
patient is incomplete, because the patient's critical condition creates a
situation where every minute counts and injuries are simply repaired as
they are encountered. Under these circumstances you must complete the
exploration before terminating the procedure.

Finally, *first do not harm*. This applies everywhere in medicine but is of
paramount importance during abdominal exploration. The injured or
infected contents of the peritoneal cavity may be inflamed, swollen,
adherent, friable and brittle. Careless and sloppy manipulation and separation of viscera during exploration commonly induce additional bleeding and may produce additional bowel defects, or enlarge the existing
ones. As usual, new problems translate into additional therapies and
morbidity.

**This is what makes emergency abdominal surgery so exciting
and demanding: the ever looming surprises and the anxiety
about whether you are able, or not, to tackle it competently.**

10 Peritonitis: Contamination and Infection – Principles of Treatment

In peritonitis-source control is above all

The finding of bowel contents or pus, localized or dispersed, throughout the peritoneal cavity is common at emergency laparotomy. How is this scenario best handled? The chapter will discuss the general aspects of the surgical treatment.

Nomenclature

Peritonitis and *intra-abdominal infection* are not synonymous. The former may result from sterile inflammation of the peritoneum, like the chemical peritonitis seen following an early perforation of a peptic ulcer or acute pancreatitis. Intra-abdominal infection implies inflammation of the peritoneum caused by microorganisms. Because, in clinical practice, the vast majority of cases of peritonitis are bacterial, these two terms are used interchangeably.

As a Reminder

- *Primary peritonitis* is caused by microorganisms, which originate from a source outside the abdomen. In young girls, it is usually a *Streptococcus* gaining access via the genital tract; in cirrhotics, *E.Coli* is thought to be a blood-borne agent infecting the ascites; and in patients receiving peritoneal dialysis, *Staphylococcus* migrates from the skin along the dialysis catheter. Primary peritonitis in patients without a predisposing factor, such as ascites or dialysis catheter, is extremely rare. It is usually diagnosed during a laparotomy for an 'acute abdomen" when odorless pus is found without an apparent source. The diagnosis is reached by exclusion (after a thorough abdominal exploration) and is confirmed by a Gram-stain and culture, which document a solitary organism. In patients with a known pre-disposing factor (e.g. ascites) primary peritonitis should be suspected and diagnosed by paracentesis, thus avoiding an operation. Treatment is with antibiotics, initially empiric, until results of bacteriological sensitivities become available.

- *Secondary peritonitis* implies that the source of infection is a disrupted or inflamed abdominal viscus. This entity is the "bread and butter" for you, the general surgeon.
- *Tertiary peritonitis* (see chapter 38)
- *Intra-abdominal infection* (IAI) is defined as an inflammatory response of the peritoneum to microorganisms and their toxins that results in a purulent exudate in the abdominal cavity.
- *Abdominal contamination* represents conditions without a significant peritoneal inflammatory response: soiling has occurred but infection is not established yet (e.g. early traumatic bowel perforation).
- *Resectable IAI* represents infectious processes that are contained within a diseased but resectable organ (e.g. gangrenous appendicitis). These conditions are easily eradicated by an operation and consequently – do not require prolonged postoperative antibiotic therapy.
- *Non-resectable IAI* are infections which have spread beyond the confines of the source-organ. In perforated appendicitis, for instance, you may resect the appendix but residual peritoneal infection persists, requiring extended antibiotic coverage.
- *Abdominal sepsis* is still a term used very commonly, yet it is confusing. According to modern consensus "sepsis" means systemic inflammatory response syndrome (SIRS) plus a source of infection (chapter 38). The use of "sepsis", in the abdominal context, would not take into account the important initial *local* inflammation

within the peritoneal cavity. This peritoneal response is analogous, 69
at a local level, with SIRS at the systemic level, as it represents, likewise, a nonspecific inflammatory response of the host to a variety
of noxious stimuli, not necessarily infectious. Strictly speaking,
therefore, *local contamination, infection and sepsis refer to different
processes.* Yet, they may co-exist in the same patient, developing
simultaneously or consecutively. The soiling of the peritoneal cavity
with feces may result in one or other pathological entity, belonging
to a continuum of local and systemic conditions, ranging from local
contamination to septic shock. Untreated or neglected abdominal
contamination progresses to intra-abdominal infection, which is
invariably associated with a systemic inflammatory response. More
significantly, abdominal inflammation or indeed the systemic
response (fever, leukocytosis) may even persist after the intra-
peritoneal infection has been eradicated.

This is not just semantic hair-splitting. It has indeed clinical relevance in
practical management situations. *Abdominal contamination* is controlled
by the local peritoneal defense mechanisms, assisted by operative peritoneal toilet and *prophylactic* antibiotics. *Resectable infection* is managed
by the resection of the contained focus of infection, supplemented with a
short *peri-operative* course of antibiotics. Infection, which is not entirely
'resectable', requires surgical control of its source; in this situation,
therapeutic antibiotics are continued postoperatively (chapters 6 & 32).

Management

The outcome of an intra-abdominal infection (IAI) depends on the
virulence of infection, the patient's pre-morbid reserves and his physiological compromise. Your goal here is to assist the patient's own local
and systemic defenses.

70   *The philosophy of management* is simple. It revolves around *control* and comprises two steps: *source* control, followed by *damage* control.

Source Control

The sine qua non-of success is timely surgical intervention to stop delivery of bacteria and adjuvants of inflammation (e.g. bile, blood, fecal fiber, barium) into the peritoneal cavity. All other measures are of little use if the operation does not successfully eradicate the infective source and reduce the inoculum to an amount that can be handled effectively by the patient's defenses supported by antibiotic therapy. This is not controversial; the rest may be.

Source control frequently involves a simple procedure such as appendectomy (chapter 22) or closure of a perforated ulcer (chapter 13). Occasionally, a major resection to remove the infective focus is indicated, such as gastrectomy or colectomy, for perforated gastric carcinoma (chapter 13) or colonic diverticulitis (chapter 23), respectively. Generally, the choice of the procedure, and whether the ends of resected bowel are anastomosed or exteriorized (creation of a stoma), depends on the anatomical source of infection, the degree of peritoneal inflammation and SIRS, and the patient's pre morbid reserves, as will be discuss in the individual chapters.

Damage Control

This comprises maneuvers aimed at cleaning the peritoneal cavity; in bodily terms – a "*peritoneal toilet*". What should it entail?

Contaminants and infectious fluids should be aspirated and particulate matter removed by swabbing or mopping the peritoneal surfaces with moist laparotomy pads. Although cosmetically appealing and popular with surgeons, there is no evidence that *intra-operative peritoneal lavage* reduces mortality or infective complications in patients receiving adequate systemic

antibiotics. Also *peritoneal irrigation with antibiotics* is not advantageous,   71
and the addition of antiseptics may produce toxic effects. You may use
"copious irrigation" as much as you wish but know that beyond wetting
your own underwear and shoes, you do not accomplish much. Should
you choose to remain a dedicated irrigator remember to suck out all the
lavage fluid before you close; there is evidence that leaving saline or Ringer's
behind interferes with peritoneal defenses by "diluting the macrophages".
Bacteria swim perhaps better than macrophages!

The concept of *radical debridement of the peritoneal cavity*, by removing every bit of fibrin, which covers the peritoneal surfaces and viscera,
did not withstand the test of a prospective randomized study, as aggressive
debridement causes excessive bleeding from the denuded peritoneum
and endangers the integrity of the friable intestine.

Despite the *dictum that it is impossible to effectively drain the free
peritoneal cavity*, drains are still commonly used and misused. Their use
should be limited to the evacuation of an established abscess, to allow
escape of potential visceral secretions (e.g., biliary, pancreatic) and,
rarely, to establish a controlled intestinal fistula when the latter cannot
be exteriorize. To prevent erosion of intestine use soft drains, for the
shortest duration possible, keeping it away from bowel. In general,
active-suction drainage is better than the passive, and infective complications can be reduced using "closed "systems. Drains provide a false
sense of security and reassurance; we have all seen the moribund postoperative patient with an abdomen "crying" to be re-explored while his
surgeon strongly denying any possibility of intra-peritoneal catastrophe
because the tiny drains he inserted, in each abdominal quadrant, are
"dry" and non-productive.

The role of *postoperative peritoneal lavage*, through tube drains,
which were left behind, is at best questionable. The basic question
remains whether it is possible to irrigate the whole abdominal cavity, as
tubes or drains are rapidly 'walled-off' by adhesions and adjacent tissues.
You'll be irrigating nothing more than the drains' tract.

Aggressive Modalities of Management

In combination with competent supportive management and appropriate antibiotic administration most of your IAI patients will respond to the aforementioned steps. Most but not all: a few will need more. During the 1980's it became clear that if the initial standard operation fails, persisting or recurrent IAI sometimes is overlooked or the diagnosis is delayed. Waiting for signs of persisting infection or organ failure as the indication for re-exploration ('on demand') of the abdomen often proves futile. To improve results, two new concepts of *aggressive management* had to be addressed: to *repeat or ascertain source control* and to *extend damage control*:

- *Planned re-laparotomy* – this continues the process of source control: multiple operative interventions are planned before or during (but not after) the first procedure for peritonitis. The commitment is made to return to the abdominal cavity to re-explore, evacuate, debride or resect as needed, until those disease processes are resolved (chapter 37).

- *Open management (laparostomy)* – as an addition to damage control it facilitates frequent re-explorations. It serves to decompress the high intra-abdominal pressure caused by peritoneal edema associated with inflammation and fluid resuscitation, thus obviating the deleterious systemic consequences of the *abdominal compartment syndrome* (chapter 28 & 37).

Early results of these methods were promising, particularly in the management of infected pancreatic necrosis but were less favorable in cases of postoperative peritonitis, perhaps because the sickest patients were included. Intestinal fistulas plagued simple open management – problems which were almost eliminated by introduction of *temporary abdominal closure* (TAC) techniques as explained in chapter 37. Our indications to pursue with these modalities are as following:

- Critical patients condition (hemodynamic instability) precluding appropriate source control at the first operation.
- Excessive peritoneal (visceral) swelling preventing abdominal closure without excessive tension.
- Massive abdominal wall loss.
- Impossibility to eliminate or to control the source of infection.
- Incomplete debridement of necrotic tissue.
- Uncertainty of viability of remaining bowel (chapter 19).
- Uncontrolled bleeding (the need for 'packing').

In our experience, a minority (remember, we promised not to use percentages) of all patients operated upon for IAI will qualify for such management modalities. Note also that such aggressive treatment methods have increased risk of complications associated with its use. The possibility has been raised that re-laparotomies constitute a "second hit" in patients in whom the inflammatory response is already "switched-on" – thus escalating the systemic inflammatory response syndrome (SIRS)- (chapter 38). To solve this controversy, prospective randomized studies are necessary but extremely difficult, if not impossible, to organize. We believe, however, that these techniques are beneficial if initiated early, in well-selected patients, for specific indications, and performed by a team of dedicated surgeons. Conversely, an indiscriminate use, at "the end of the operative list", often by ever changing members of junior staff, represent a recipe for disasters (chapter 37).

Intra-abdominal Abscess

Many surgical texts still, erroneously, use the term intra-abdominal abscess as a synonym with peritonitis. This is not true as abscesses develop due to effective host defenses and represent a relatively successful outcome of peritonitis. *The mainstay of treatment is drainage, but by which route?* This is discussed in details in chapter 35.

Need for Peritoneal Cultures

The expensive ritual of obtaining routine, intra-operative peritoneal cultures has become questionable. Think, how many times did you act, changing antibiotics, based on peritoneal culture results? Probably, never! As you saw above, the microbiology of IAI is predictable, the pathogens being 'covered' by the broad-spectrum empiric agents started by you prior to the operation (chapter 6). Furthermore, usually after a few days, when culture and sensitivity results are available, the antibiotics are no longer necessary. Being a modern surgeon you stopped them at the appropriate time (chapter 32). Recently we conducted an audit among Infection Disease (ID) specialists and a group of surgeons interested in surgical infections. We asked them the following question: a patient undergoes a laparotomy three hours after receiving a gunshot injury to his abdomen. At operation you find a hole in the left colon and fecal peritoneal contamination. Would you send the peritoneal fluid for culture and sensitivity?

Guess what was the response? Almost all (95%) of the ID specialists would have send the pure feces for culture – as if they do not know what kind bacteria it contains! But now you know better then them: you know that the discussed patient had peritoneal contamination – necessitating source control, peritoneal toilet and prophylactic peri-operative antibiotics. Nothing more!

Shakiness of the hand may be some bar to the successful performance of an operation, but he of a shaky mind is hopeless (Sir Macewen)

11 The Intestinal Anastomosis

The enemy of good is better: the first layer is the best – why spoil it?

The Ideal Anastomosis

The ideal intestinal anastomosis is the one, which does not leak, for leaks, although relatively rare, represent a dreaded and deadly disaster (chapter 39). In addition, the anastomosis should not obstruct, allowing normally functioning gastrointestinal tract within a few days of construction.

Any experienced surgeon thinks that his anastomotic technique, adopted from his mentors and with a touch of personal virtuosity, is the "best". Many methods are practiced: end-to-end, end-to-side or side-to-side; single versus double layered, interrupted versus continuous, using absorbable versus non-absorbable, braided versus monofilament, suture materials. We even know some obsessive surgeons who carefully construct a 3-layers anastomosis in an interrupted fashion. To this variability add staplers. So where do we stand; what is preferable?

Pro & Cons

Numerous experimental and clinical studies support the following:
- *Leakage*: the incidence of anastomotic dehiscence is identical-irrespective of the method used, provided the anastomosis is technically sound: constructed with well-perfused bowel and without tension and being water and air tight.
- *Stricture*: the single-layer anastomosis is associated with a lower incidence of stricture formation than the multi-layered one. Strictures are also commoner following end-to end-anastomosis performed with the circular stapler.

- *Misadventure*: overall, staplers are more prone to intra-operative technical failures or "misfires".
- *Speed*: stapled anastomoses, on the average, are slightly faster than that sutured by hand. The fewer are the layers – the faster is the anastomosis and the continuous method is swifter than the interrupted one. Conceptually, the time consumed to place 2 'purse-string' sutures for a stapled circular anastomosis is identical to that required to complete a hand sutured, single-layered, continuous anastomosis.
- *Suture material*: braided sutures (e.g. silk or vicryl) 'saw' through tissues and, experimentally at least, are associated with greater inflammation and activation of collagenases, than monofilament material (e.g. PDS, proline). 'Chromic catgut' is too rapidly absorbed to support (alone) an anastomosis. Monofilament slides better through the tissues and, when used in a continuous fashion, is self-adjustable to equally distribute the tension along the entire circumference of the anastomosis.
- *Cost*: staplers are much more expensive than sutures and, thus, generally not cost-effective. Because the less suture material is used the cheaper is the anastomosis, single layer – continuous technique is more economical.

The Choice of Anastomotic Technique

Since all methods, if correctly performed, are safe, nobody can fault you for using the anastomotic method which you are most familiar and comfortable with. We maintain, however, and we may be biased, that the one-layer, continuous method, using a monofilament suture material, is the one a "modern surgeon" should adopt, because it is fast, cheap and safe. What is good for the high-pressure vascular anastomosis should be as good for the low-pressure intestinal one. If the first layer suffices – why

narrow and injure it with another one of inverted and strangulated
tissue? Would you replace a well-done hamburger on the grill?

We acknowledge that staplers are elegant, "admired" by the nursing
operating room staff, "fun" to use and of great financial benefit to its
manufactures. Certainly, staples may be advantageous in selected problematic, rectal or esophageal anastomoses, deep in the pelvis or high
under the diaphragm. But those types of anastomoses are rarely performed
in emergency situations. Furthermore, as a surgical trainee you should
start using the staplers only after achieving maximal proficiency in manual
techniques, and in difficult circumstances. Even the stapler aficionado
has to use his hands when the instrument misfires, or cannot be used
because of specific anatomic constrain such as the retroperitoneal
duodenum. The modern surgeon and the trainee too, need to be equally
proficient in hand-sewn and stapled anastomosis; we suggest, however,
that before driving a car you learn to ride a bicycle.

The Edematous Bowel

It is our experience that continuous monolayer anastomosis occasionally
fails when performed in *edematous bowel* (e.g. after massive fluid resuscitation, severe peritonitis). From findings at re-operation we learned
that subsequently, as the bowel edema subsides, the suture may become
loose, leading to anastomotic dehiscence. Therefore, when anastomosing
swollen bowel we prefer to use a closely placed layer of interrupted
sutures. We admit, however, that scientific data to back this hypothesis is
lacking.

78   Technique

Our preferred – continuous, monolayered anastomosis uses one double-armed, or two regular, 3–0 or 4–0 monofilament sutures (PDS or maxon). No bowel clamps are used, as we like to assess the adequacy of blood supply to the bowel edges. It is not necessary to devascularize the bowel edges by "cleaning off" the fat at the mesenteric side or removing appendices epiploica. The suture line begins at the posterior wall, running "over and over" towards both sides to meet, and be tied, anteriorly. The secret is to take generous bites through the submucosa, muscularis and serosa and avoid the mucosa ("big bites outside, small bites inside"). The needle exit or entry site on the serosal side is at least 5–7 mm from the bowel edge while the distance between the bites should be such as not to allow access to the tips of a Debakey forceps (3–4 mm). The assistant who "follows" with the suture should maintain only a moderate tension in order not to strangulate the tissue. Identical technique suits the end to side or side to side versions and, in essence, it is the intestinal version of a routine vascular anastomosis. We use the above technique throughout the entire gastrointestinal tract, from the esophagus above – down to the rectum. Essentially, you create a wide lumen, inverted, and safe anastomosis, using a suture or two, in less than 15 minutes.

In "difficult" situations – when the anastomotic site is relatively inaccessible – we prefer a one-layer interrupted technique, which allow a more accurate placement of sutures. 'How to do' the latter and how to correctly use the stapler you will learn from your mentors.

Testing the Anastomosis

A correctly performed anastomosis – when indicated – should not leak. There is no point to routinely test your "routine" intra-abdominal intestinal anastomosis; the common practice of pinching-masturbating the anastomosis to confirm an adequate lumen is laughable if you used a one-layer technique as described above. "Problematic" anastomoses such, as those performed to the distal rectum should be tested: simply clamp the bowel above the anastomosis, fill the pelvis with saline and inject air into the rectum. Instead of air you may wish to use dye. When air bubbles or dye are observed leaking; attempt to correct the defect; if unsuccessful – a proximal diverting stoma is indicated.

When Not To Perform an Anastomosis?

We wish we had an exact answer! In broad terms, whenever the probability for a future leak is high – avoid an anastomosis since anastomotic leak usually implies disastrous consequences. But how do you accurately predict anastomotic failure?

Traditionally, the avoidance of colonic suture line during emergency operation for trauma, obstruction, or perforation was the established practice. But, times are changing; whereas during WW II a colostomy was mandatory for any colonic injury, currently we successfully repair most such wounds (chapter 27). Furthermore, three – or two-stage procedures for colonic obstruction are being replaced by the one-stage resection-anastomosis (chapter 21).

It is difficult to lay down precise guidelines as to when an intestinal anastomosis is not to be made. You should make a careful decision after considering *the condition of the patient, the intestine, and the peritoneal cavity*. Generally, we would avoid a colonic anastomosis in the presence of established and diffuse intra-abdominal infection (as opposed to contamination) (chapter 23). Regarding the small bowel, anastomosis is indicated in most instances; however, when more than one of the following factors are present we tend to err on the conservative side and exteriorize or divert, depending on technical circumstances.

80
- Postoperative peritonitis (chapter 37)
- Leaking anastomosis (chapter 39)
- Mesenteric ischemia (chapter 19)
- Extreme bowel edema/distention (chapter 28)
- Extreme malnutrition (chapter 31)
- Chronic steroids intake
- Unstable patient (damage control situation) (chapter 27)

No formula or algorithm are available, so use your judgement but try not be too obsessive to always try to anastomose. Yes, we know that you wish the patient well by wanting to spare him a stoma, but please try not to kill him. You should not be fearful of creating a high small bowel stoma. The latter was previously considered unmanageable. Today, however, with TPN, techniques of distal enteric re-feeding, somatostatin, and stoma care, these temporary proximal intestinal "vents" can be life saving (see also chapter 31). For anastomotic leaks see chapter 39.

Conclusions

The intestinal anastomosis is the "elective" part of the emergency operation you are going to perform. Remember – your aim is to save life and minimize morbidity; create an anastomosis when its chances to succeed are at least reasonable. There are many ways to skin a cat and fashion an anastomosis. Master a few methods and use them selectively.

12 Upper Gastrointestinal Hemorrhage

> – *When the blood is fresh and pink and the patient is old,*
>   *it is time to be active and bold.*
> – *When the patient is young and the blood is dark and old,*
>   *you can relax and put your knife on hold*

The way surgeons consider acute upper gastrointestinal hemorrhage (UGI-H) has been modified over recent years by the following factors:

- Due to the availability of modern anti-ulcer pharmacological therapy the incidence of active and poorly controlled peptic ulcers is declining.
- The introduction of anti-Helicobacter therapy has reduced the incidence of ulcer's recurrence.
- The availability of methods to achieve trans-endoscopic hemostasis of bleeding ulcers.
- Consequently, you are becoming less and less familiar and skilled with the operative management of this condition. Therefore, you need to listen to us ...

The Problem

UGI-H implies a source *proximal to the ligament of Treitz*. Although textbooks list multiple causes, the vast majority of patients bleed from a chronic duodenal (DU) and gastric (GU) ulcers, complications of portal hypertension (esophageal varices or hypertensive gastropathy), or acute gastric mucosal lesions (e.g. stress ulcers, erosive gastritis and other terms which mean more or less the same). The latter are usually due to ingestion of analgesics or/with alcohol ("aspirin for the hangover"). With the routine use of anti-ulcer prophylaxis in the hospitalized 'stressed' patients, significant UGI-H from mucosal lesions has become uncommon.

82   In fact, hemorrhage in 'stressed' patients often originates from re-activated chronic peptic ulcers. The admixture of etiologies in your hospital depends on local social habits and the sort of population you work with.

Presentation

Patients present either with *hematemesis* (vomiting fresh blood), *melenemesis* (vomiting altered "coffee-ground) or *melena* (passage of black stool per rectum). *Hematochezia* (passage of fresh or altered non-black blood per rectum) usually originates from a source below the ligament of Treitz. Nevertheless, with massive UGI-H, and rapid intestinal transit, unaltered blood may appear in the rectum.

Remember

- Black blood per rectum means always UGI bleeding.
- Fresh-red blood per rectum in a hemodynamically stable patient means that the source is NOT at the UGI tract.
- Any type of blood – fresh or old – vomited or retrieved through the nasogastric tube- means that the source is at the UGI tract.

You do not need pan-endoscopy to diagnose an UGI-H –as gastroenterologists often like to do. A finger, a nasogastric tube and set of eyes are as good.

Key Issue: Is the Hemorrhage "Serious"?

This is a key issue as the "seriousness" of hemorrhage determines your diagnostic-therapeutic steps and patients' outcome. In general, the larger

the bleeding vessel, the more "serious" is the hemorrhage. The more
"serious" is the hemorrhage, the less likely it is to stop without your
intervention or to recur after it has stopped. As with almost any acute
medical or surgical condition the affected patients can be allocated into
three groups. The obviously "serious" and obviously "not serious" on
both extremes, and the "potentially serious" group in the middle. The
"intermediate" group is always the most problematic in terms of diagnosis
and selection of therapy but, at the same time, includes those patients in
whom your correct management can improve outcome. Whatever the
condition is, the mildly ill patient should do well, the very sick one may
die in spite of your efforts; your intervention has most to offer in the
moderately ill.

Patient Stratification

Massive bleeding from a large vessel requires your immediate attention
and intervention; it may stop but will commonly recur. Small ooze from
a tiny vessel is usually self-limited and of minor significant at least for
the moment; you can further investigate it electively. For most patients,
seeing any quantity of blood emerging from any orifice is alarming.

When Should You Be Alarmed?

The literature contains various formulas, usually based on hemodynamic
parameters and the volume of blood transfusions required, to distinguish
between massive versus non-massive UGI-H. We suggest, however, that
you use your clinical judgement and consider the clinical paradigm
consisting of the following:
*   Was the vomited blood (or appearing in the NG tube) fresh or
     "coffee ground"?

84
- Was the passed stool, or found on rectal examination, fresh, juicy melena, or old dry melena?
- Was, or is, the patient hemodynamically compromised?
- Is there any laboratory evidence of severe bleeding (hemoglobin/hematocrit)?
- To the above add the patient's age: *bleeding in elderly patients (defined as over 60 years old) should be considered as "more serious"* because they are less likely to withstand a prolonged hemorrhage. We find the APACHE II scoring system (chapter 5) useful also in this situation as it captures the severity of bleeding, patient's physiological compromise, age and pre-existing systemic conditions.

The aforementioned consideration should place your patients within a large spectrum of UGI-H "seriousness". On one extreme, the patient presenting in shock, and with fresh blood pouring from his stomach, belongs to the *"serious" group (group I)*; on the other, the stable patient, with a little coffee ground and old dry melena is definitively *"not serious"* (group III). Many patients, however, belong to the *"potentially serious" (group II)*; the problem here is to distinguish between those who continue to 'ooze" or will re-bleed and those who stopped bleeding and their chance to re-bleed is low. This distinction requires active observation and endoscopy.

Approach

Check vital signs. The aggressive management of hypovolemic shock is the first priority. Do not over transfuse; there is good evidence that excessive blood product administration exacerbates the bleeding and results in a higher incidence of re-bleeding.

With resuscitation underway, history is taken: previous peptic ulceration? dyspepsia? anti-ulcer medications? (Remember, bleeding

patients do not have pain because blood is alkaline and serves as an 85
anti-acid). Recent analgesics or alcohol consumption? Severe vomiting or
retching (Mallory Weiss)? Nose bleed (swallowed blood)? Coagulopathy?
Amount of blood vomited or passed per rectum (extremely inaccurate)?
Full medical history (operative risk factors)?

Pass a large bore nasogastric tube, flush the stomach with 50 ml of
saline, and aspirate: fresh blood indicates active or a very recent hemorrhage; coffee ground – recent bleeding which stopped; clean aspirate or
bile – no recent hemorrhage. *Note*: rarely, a bleeding DU is associated with
a pyloric spasm with no blood refluxing into the stomach; bile-stained
aspirate excludes such a possibility.

Perform a rectal examination: fresh blood or juicy soft melena
indicates an active or very recent bleeding while dry and solid melena
signifies a non-recent UGI-H.

Now, with all the above information in your mind you can classify
the patients into one of the 3 groups (table 12.1) and proceed as following:

The "non-serious bleeder" (group III). These patients suffered a minor
hemorrhage, which stopped. Do not rush them for an endoscopy in the
middle of the night. Semi-elective investigation suffices, and is more

Table 12.1. Stratification and management of patients with upper gastrointestinal hemorrhage.

	Group I Not serious	Group II Potentially serious	Group III Serious
Vomiting	Nothing / coffee ground	Coffee ground or fresh	Fresh blood
Per rectum	Old melena	Fresh melena	Fresh melena/blood
Hemodynamically	Stable	Stable	Compromised
Hemoglobin/crit	>9/27		<9/27
Approach	Endoscopy tomorrow	Endoscopy soon	Endoscopy now
Prognosis	Self limiting	variable	Requires hemostasis

86   accurate and safer. Note that a very low hematocrit/hemoglobin in patients belonging to this group results from a chronic or intermittent "ooze". The very anemic patient will tolerate endoscopy better after his general condition is improved. Because these patients never require an *emergency* operation they won't be discussed further.

The "serious" bleeders (group I). In a minority of patients belonging to this group fresh blood is pouring torrentially from the stomach; they are virtually *exanguinating*. You have to move fast. Esophageal or gastric varices often bleed this way – as an "open tap". Previous history of portal hypertension or clinical stigmata of chronic liver disease commonly coexists, suggesting the diagnosis. *Remember: you do not want to operate on varices as an emergency.* Combining drugs (e.g. vasopressin, soma-tostatin), variceal injection- sclerotherapy or banding and, if necessary, balloon tamponade, should arrest the acute variceal hemorrhage in most instances. Be it as it may, you should transfer the exanguinating patient to a critical care facility or the operating room. *Intubate and sedate* him/her to facilitate gastric lavage and subsequent endoscopy, and, most importantly, to prevent *aspiration* in the shocked obtunded bleeding patient. You should attempt endoscopy even if gastroduodenal visualization is totally obscured by blood as fresh bleeding from the esophageal varices, (usually at 40 cm' from the teeth – the gastroesophageal junction) can be always detected, indicating a non-operative approach. In the absence of varices proceed to surgery. The "serious" patients who are not exanguina-ting should undergo an emergency endoscopy as discussed below.

The "potentially serious" bleeder (group II): Perform an emergency endoscopy.

Emergency Endoscopy for UGI-H

This should be done only after you have resuscitated the patient and in a controlled environment. Endoscopy induces hypoxemia and vagal stimu-

lation; we witnessed it causing cardiac arrest in unstable and poorly   87
oxygenated patients. *Ideally, you – the surgeon – should be the one who is
performing the procedure.* Unfortunately, because of "political" and
fiscal considerations, in many hospitals you are denied this experience
and access to the endoscope. If this is the case – be at least present at the
endoscopy to visualize, first hand, the findings. Do not entirely trust the
gastroenterologist; he'll be going home soon, leaving you with the
patient and the problems resulting from poorly identified bleeding site.

To improve the diagnostic yield the stomach should be prepared
for endoscopy. Pass the largest nasogastric tube you can find and flush
the stomach rapidly and repeatedly, aspirating as many clots as possible.
A common ritual is to use ice-cold saline (with or without vasoconstricting
agent) for this purpose. None of these methods has been proven as
therapeutic. Tap water, however, is just as good, much cheaper, and does
not aggravate hypothermia.

At endoscopy you attempt to visualize the source of bleeding which
may be esophageal (varices, Mallory-Weiss), gastric (chronic GU or superficial lesions), duodenal (DU), solitary (chronic ulcer) or multiple (erosive
gastritis). Look also for the following "stigmata":
- Active bleeding from lesion/s.
- A "visible vessel" 'standing up' at the ulcer's base, indicating that
  the bleeding originated from a large vessel and that there is a high
  chance for further hemorrhage.
- A clot adherent to the ulcer's base, signifying a recent hemorrhage.

You may like to classify the findings as following:

No evidence of recent bleeding	Evidence of recent bleeding	Active bleeding
Clean base	Flat spot	oozing
	Adherent clot	spurting
	Visible vessel	

88   Endoscopic Management

Having visualized the lesion you should now treat it endoscopically in order to achieve hemostasis and to prevent further hemorrhage. In broad terms, endoscopic therapy has a better chance to succeed in shallow lesions, which contain small vessels. You should attempt, however, endoscopic hemostasis also in deeper, large vessel-containing lesions, with the aim of achieving at least temporary cessation of bleeding. This will permit a safer, elective – definitive operation to be performed in a better-prepared patient. The specific method of endoscopic hemostasis, be it a "hot" probe or injection with adrenaline or a sclerosant, depends on local skills and facilities, and is out of the scope of these pages.

Post-endoscopy Decision Making

At the end of endoscopy you are left with the following categories of patients:
- *Actively bleeding* – failed endoscopic hemostasis. The source is usually a chronic ulcer and emergency operation is indicated.
- *Bleeding stopped*; chronic ulcer with a "visible vessel" or adherent clot visualized. The chances of further hemorrhage, usually within 48–72 hours, are substantial. Treat conservatively but *observe closely*!
- *Bleeding stopped*; acute shallow lesion or chronic ulcer without the aforementioned "stigmata". In these patients further hemorrhage is unlikely; treat conservatively and *relax*.

Conservative Treatment

The mainstay of conservative treatment comprises of completion and maintenance of resuscitative measures and watch for further hemorrhage.

Neither gastric lavage nor medications will change the acute course in   89
the individual patient. The acid-reducing medications you administer do
not reduce the incidence of early re-bleeding, and are prescribed for the
healing of ulcer in long term. Obviously, correct coagulopathies if present.
All you need to do is to sustain the patient's organ systems, and watch
for re-bleeding, which usually occurs within 48–72 hours and can be
massive and lethal. A nasogastric tube on suction is advocated to provide
early warning. In our experience, however, it is often blocked by clots, is
of great discomfort to the patient and therefore not routinely necessary.
If you chose to use it, flush it frequently. Careful monitoring of vital signs,
observation of the number and character of melena stools and serial
hematocrit measurements will detect episodes of further hemorrhage.

Indications for Operation

We do not suggest that you use cookbook recipes or formulas, as they
are of little help in the individual patient. Instead, use clinical judgement.
That the exanguinating patient, and the one who continues to bleed after
endoscopic hemostasis fails, needs an emergency operation, is clear and
has been discussed above. Regarding those in whom the hemorrhage
stopped, with or without endoscopic hemostasis, the main indication for
operation is a *recurrent hemorrhage*. Factors, which may or may not modify
your decision to operate include the magnitude of recurrent hemorrhage,
it's source, and the age and general condition of the patient. In general
terms, *recurrent hemorrhage is an ominous sign*, meaning that bleeding will
continue or, if stopped again, will re-occur! If hemodynamically significant
or originating from a chronic ulcer *you have to operate*! If re-bleeding
seems of mild or moderate magnitude and stems from a superficial lesion
you may elect to continue conservative treatment or re-treat endoscopically.
But, whatever you do remember that old and chronically ill patients poorly
tolerate repeated episodes of bleeding; *do not mess them around.*

90   Operative Management

Repeat Endoscopy

It is crucial that you know from where in the UGI the patient is bleeding. If the initial endoscopy was not done by you, or in your presence, *do it again*. In an anesthetized patient it will not take you more than 5 minutes to insert and remove the endoscope. Do not trust the written, 2 days old endoscopic's report, that the "source of hemorrhage appeared to be in the duodenum". It may lead to an unnecessary duodenotomy while the source lies high in the stomach.

Exploration

An upper midline incision, supplemented with a para- xyphoid extension and forceful upwards sternal retraction, lets you deal with anything in the forgut. In obese, wide costal angle, patients, however, a transverse-chevron type incision, make take a few more minutes, but affords a more comfortable exposure. In addition, a *generous reverse-Trendelenburg tilt of the patient will bring the upper stomach almost into your nose.*

Start by searching for external visual or palpable features of chronic ulceration. The latter are invariably associated with serosal inflammatory changes. Look for evidence of chronic ulcers from the duodenum to the gastric cardia. Duodenal Kocherization will be necessary to reveal the sporadic postbulbar ulcer in the second portion of the duodenum. Occasionally, a posterior or lesser curvature GU will become palpable only through the lesser sac. Acute superficial mucosal lesions are unfortunately not identifiable from the outside although a Mallory Weiss lesion may be tattooed by bluish serosal staining at the gastroesophageal junction.

The finding of a chronic ulcer in accordance with the pre-operative
endoscopic finding tells you where the trouble is; but what to do in the
absence of any external evidence of pathology? You have a few options:

- Proceed according to the endoscopic findings but occasionally
  they are not definitive.
- Surgical exploration.
- Intra-operative endoscopy.

Intra-operative Endoscopy

Having endoscopically visualized, with your own eyes, an actively bleeding
DU, you should not have any doubts. A doubtful endoscopic report,
however, may promote a negative duodenotomy, extending it – piecemeal –
proximally, until the acute high gastric lesion is found. All what was
needed was a small high gastrotomy and suture ligation of the lesion;
instead you are left with a very long and unnecessary duodenogastrotomy
defect to repair. To obviate such a mini-disaster we would unscrub for a
moment and "shove" in an endoscope through the mouth. Commonly,
when the stomach is distended with huge clots, we would place a purse-
string suture at the anterior wall of the antrum; perform a small gastrotomy;
and with a large sucker remove and irrigate all clots. An endoscope is
than inserted through the gastrotomy with the purse-string tightened
to allow gastric insufflation; this offers excellent and controlled view of
the stomach and duodenum. We call it: intra-operative retrograde
gastroscopy.

Philosophy of Surgical Management

*The general philosophy here is that saving lives, namely, stopping the bleeding,
comes first.* This is the main consideration in the severely ill patients. In

92   the less compromised subjects, *the secondary issue of long term cure of disease may be considered*. Although most surgeons accept this straightforward philosophy the methods they use to accomplish it are fiercely debated. We suggest that you select the operative approach based on the following:

- Do the minimum necessary in the severely ill (e.g. APACHE II >10)
- In the "fit" patients (e.g. APACHE II <10) tailor the definitive anti-ulcer procedure to the ulcer-type and patient.
- Gastric resection is usually *not* necessary to provide secure hemostasis or/and long-term cure.

Specific Sources of Bleeding

Duodenal Ulcer (DU)

The source of bleeding is always at the base of a posterior ulcer. Hemostasis is accomplished through an anterior duodenotomy, underrunning the base (and bleeding vessel) with 2–3 (2–0 monofilament) deeply placed sutures – each placed in a different "direction". When bleeding is active the successful ligation of the vessel will be evident; in it's absence you may want to 'rub a little' the ulcer's base, dislodging the clot and inducing bleeding. Otherwise, just underrun the base; deeply, and in a few directions. *The theoretical danger of underrunning a nearby common bile duct has been mentioned but not even one such a case has been ever reported.* After achieving hemostasis you are left with a few options. In the very compromised patient all you want is to stop the bleeding; close the duodenotomy without constricting the lumen and get out; leaving the eventual cure of the ulcer to acid or/and Helicobacter – reducing drugs. In a less compromised individual you may choose to prolong the operation by 30 minutes, adding a truncal vagotomy (TV), extending the duodenotomy across the pylorus, and closing it to form a Heinke-

Mikulitz pyloroplasty. In a 'fit' and stable patient we would close the
duodenotomy and perform a highly selective vagotomy (HSV), adding
an hour or so to the procedure. Local hemostasis can be achieved even
in the base of giant ulcers or when the duodenum is extremely inflamed
or scarred; when simple closure of the duodenotmy appears to compromise the lumen or pyloroplasty deemed unsatisfactory; just close the
duodenum and add a posterior gastroenterostomy (GE) to the TV or
HSV. The proponents of antrectomy plus vagotomy for bleeding DU
claim an increased incidence of re-hemorrhage when gastric resection is
avoided. In over a hundred emergency operations for bleeding DU we
did not experience a significant re-bleeding from the sutured ulcer and
thus believe that there is no sense in removing a healthy stomach, producing gastric cripples, for a benign duodenal disease – which anyway
can be subsequently cured with medications.

Postbulbar DU

For unknown reasons this kind of ulcer has almost disappeared from the
"Western world". Although extensive resective procedures (including an
emergency Whipple's) are mentioned in the old literature, all you need
to do is to mobilize the duodenum; underrun the ulcer through a duodenotomy, and – perhaps – add a TV or a HSV and a GE.

Gastric Ulcer (GU)

Traditionally, for most surgeons, a bleeding GU mandated a partial gastrectomy. Gastric resection is indeed effective in controlling the hemorrhage,
but in most instances represents a superfluous ritual. For acute-superficial
ulcers all what is required is simple underrunning of the lesion through
a small gastrotomy. Also in the critically-ill patient who bleed from a
chronic GU simple underrunning of the ulcer from within, through a
gastrotomy, suffices. In large chronic ulcer we first underrun the bleeding

94 point with an absorbable suture; with a heavy absorbable suture we then
obliterate the ulcer's base. UGI-H from a malignant ulcer very rarely is
severe enough to require an emergency operation. We would, however,
take tissue from the ulcer's edges for histology. Partial gastrectomy becomes mandatory only in cases of a giant GU on the lesser curvature, with
direct involvement of the left gastric or splenic arteries.

After hemostasis, in 'fit' and stable patients a definitive ulcer
procedure may be considered. Chronic GU is not "one disease" to be
managed by a ritual gastrectomy; instead it comprises of different types
which should be managed selectively:

- *Type I* is the classical lesser curvature GU. Billroth I partial
gastrectomy is the "text book" recommendation. An HSV (from
the ulcer proximally) plus the excision of the ulcer (from inside
the stomach) is the alternative which we recommend instead.
- *Type II* is a pre-pyloric ulcer. Though antrectomy plus vagotomy
are popular for this "hybrid" – between DU and GU – ulcer,
excellent results are achieved with HSV plus pyloroplasty. This is
what we do.
- *Type III* is a combination of a GU and a DU; it should be treated as
type II.
- *Type IV* implies a high, juxta-cardial lesser curvature GU. Prior to
the days of effective anti-ulcer medication partial gastrectomy, distal
to the ulcer, was the procedure of choice. Since the entire lesser
curvature may be obliterated, HSV is usually impossible – making
TV plus a drainage procedure a reasonable alternative. *"Riding"*
GU is a variant of a high GU associated with sliding hiatal hernia,
produced by injury to the herniated stomach "riding" against the
diaphragm. Surgical therapy involves reduction of the stomach by
pinching the ulcer away from the adherent diaphragm, local hemostasis, and crural repair. This may be, however, easier said than
done since occasionally the huge riding ulcer adheres to mediastinal
structures – requiring major resective surgery.

Stomal Ulcer

This ulcer develops on the jejunal side of the gastrojejunal anastomosis, following a previous vagotomy and GE or Billroth II gastrectomy. Because stomal ulcers almost never involve a large blood vessel, hemorrhage is usually self -limited or responsive to endoscopic therapy. Remember also that the vast majority of stomal ulcers will heal on modern acid- suppressing medications. Persisting or recurrent hemorrhage, however, will force you, rarely, to operate. In the high risk patient do the minimum: through a small gastrotomy, perpendicular to the anastomosis, examine the stoma and ulcer; underrun the later with a few deeply placed absorbable sutures; close the gastrotomy and put the patient on H-2 antagonists for life. In a better risk patient you can opt for a more definitive procedure. If the previous operation was a vagotomy plus GE- look for a missed vagal nerve or add an antrectomy. In the case of a previous Billroth II gastrectomy add TV or consider a higher gastrectomy (do not forget to rule out The Zollinger Ellison syndrome later on). Remember: at operation, hemorrhage from a stomal ulcer can be arrested with a simple surgical maneuver (underrunning); try to stay out of trouble by not escalating the emergency procedure into complicated-reconstructive gastric surgery which may kill your bleeding patient.

Delayfoey's Lesion

This small solitary and difficult to diagnose gastric vascular malformation typically causes a recurrent "obscure" massive UGI-H. It is best managed by trans-gastric excision or underrunning.

Acute Superficial Mucosal Lesions

Due to effective anti-ulcer prophylaxis in critically ill patients you will be called to operate on such lesions only a few times in your surgical life.

96   When massive hemorrhage necessitating an operation, however, occurs, the involved stomach looks and behaves as a blood- soaked and dripping sponge. Surgical options mentioned by the textbook include TV and drainage or total gastrectomy. The former is associated with a very high rate of re-bleeding and the later with a prohibitive mortality rate. In this situation we advocate *gastric devascularization by ligating the two gastro-epiploic, and left and right gastric arteries near the stomach's wall*. This, relatively simple and well tolerated procedure results in an immediate "drying of the gastric sponge".

UGI-H from an Unknown Source

You won't encounter many of those following the above suggestions, including – if necessary – the resort to intra-operative endoscopy. Angiography is an option and an excuse by those looking for a pretext to delay surgery. It is useless when performed when bleeding is not active.

Conclusions

Admit patients with UGI-H to your surgical service – not to medicine. After resuscitation diagnose the source of hemorrhage and stage it. Give endoscopic treatment a chance but do not delay an operation-if indicated. At surgery – stop the bleeding – remembering that most ulcers can be cured later on by medications. Life comes first.

13 Perforated Peptic Ulcer

There is a hole in my bucket... How should I mend it?
Just patch it! – (A folk song)

Due to the effective, modern anti-ulcer drug management the incidence of perforated peptic ulcers has decreased drastically, but not everywhere. Perforated ulcers are still common in the socio-economically disadvantaged or stressed populations, worldwide. Usually perforations develop on the background of chronic symptomatic ulceration but "denovo" presentation without previous history is not uncommon. In the "Western World" perforated duodenal ulcers (DU) are much more common than perforated gastric ulcers (GU) which are seen more in lower socioeconomic groups.

Natural History

Classically, the abdominal pain caused by a peptic perforation develops very suddenly in the upper abdomen. Most patients can accurately time the dramatic onset of symptoms. The natural history of a perforated episode can be divided into 3 phases:

*   *Chemical peritonitis/contamination.* Initially, the perforation leads to chemical peritonitis, with or without contamination with micro-organisms. (Note that the presence of acid sterilizes gastroduodenal contents; it is when gastric acid is reduced by treatment or disease – such as cancer – bacteria and fungi are present in the stomach and duodenum). Spillage of gastroduodenal contents is usually diffuse but may be localized in the upper abdomen by adhesions or the omentum. Spillage along the right gutter into the right lower quadrant, mimicking acute appendicitis, is mentioned in every textbook but almost never seen in clinical practice.

- *Intermediate stage.* After 6 to 12 hours many patients obtain some spontaneous relief of the pain. This is probably due to the dilution of the irritating gastroduodenal contents by the ensuing peritoneal exudate.
- *Intra-abdominal infection.* Should the patient escape the scalpel hitherto, after 12 to 24 hours intra-abdominal infection supervenes. The exact point in time in the individual patient when contaminating microorganisms become invasive – infective, is unknown. *Therefore, you should consider any perforation operated upon with a delay of more than 12 hours as infection rather than contamination.* This bears on your postoperative antibiotic therapy as discussed below. Neglected patients may present a few days after the perforation in septic shock. Shock in the earlier stages is very rare although quoted commonly by medical students; *but when confronted with a combination of shock and abdominal pain think about ruptured aortic aneurysm, mesenteric ischemia or severe acute pancreatitis.* Untreated perforation can lead eventually to an early 'septic' death from peritonitis or the development of an intra-abdominal abscess.

Diagnosis

The vast majority of patients present with signs of diffuse or localized peritoneal irritation; most lie still, groaning, and have a board-like abdomen "as in the textbook". Spontaneous "sealing off" of the perforation, localization of the spill, or leakage into the lesser sac, causes atypical and delayed presentation. In a patient with an abrupt onset of upper abdominal pain and diffuse peritonitis the diagnosis is simple. It can be summarized in the following *formula*:

sudden onset peritonitis+free air = perforated viscus
sudden onset peritonitis +no free air +normal amylase = perforated viscus

There is free air under the diaphragm in about two-thirds of perforated
patients. Remember, free air is visualized better on upright chest X ray
than on plain abdominal radiographs (chapter 3). If your patient won't
stand, or sit up, order a right lateral decubitus abdominal films. Free air
is diagnostic, although not always it is due to a perforated peptic ulcer.
But so what?; it signifies a perforated viscus and a laparotomy is almost
always indicated. *Beware, however, that free air without clinical peritonitis
is NOT an indication for an emergency laparotomy.* As mentioned in
chapter 3 there is a long list of "non-operative" conditions which may
produce free intra-peritoneal air such as a tension pneumothorax or
even vigorous felatio (oral sex). Free air in a "soft" abdomen may also
mean that the perforation has been spontaneously sealed and is amenable
to non-operative therapy as discussed below.

   *In the absence of free air, acute pancreatitis – the "great simulator" –
should be considered and excluded* (chapter 14). Normal serum amylase
levels support a diagnosis of a perforation while very elevated amylase
levels in a "susceptible" patient (e.g. alcohol, gallstones) suggests acute
pancreatitis. The "border line " patient with atypical presentation and
marginal elevation of amylase remains a problem (note: perforated ulcer
may cause hyperamylasemia). In the "good old days", before imaging
techniques replaced clinical skills, our decision to operate or continue to
observe would have depended on the whole clinical picture. Rarely, a
gastrografin study was performed to demonstrate or exclude free leakage.
Faced with such a patient today we would advice you to obtain a CT scan
of the abdomen, looking for free air, extraluminal gastrografin, free
peritoneal fluid and the pancreas.

Philosophy of Treatment

The *primary goal of treatment is to save the patient's life by eliminating
the source of infection and cleaning his abdominal cavity. The secondary*

goal is to cure, if possible, the ulcer-diathesis. The former goal may be achieved by simple closure of the ulcer; the latter requires a definitive ulcer operation. *When to do what?* Before telling you what to do we must answer a few other questions:

Who Are the Patients
Who Require A Definitive Procedure?

Twenty years ago the reply was simpler. The *"law of thirds"* maintained that after a simple closure of perforation one third of the patients is cured permanently, another third would require long-term medical anti-ulcer therapy, and the last third would require definitive ulcer surgery because of intractability or further complications. This provided us with a rational to add a definitive procedure in order to cure the ulcer in two-thirds of the patients. With the emergence of modern anti-ulcer agents we were told that definitive ulcer procedures are not necessary as all perforated patients could be maintained indefinitely and effectively on proper anti-ulcer drugs. Our contra-argument was then that an ulcer operation is more cost-effective than life-long commitment to drugs; that patients often are not compliant with the latter, and, in fact, often perforate while taking anti-ulcer drugs. Now, with the availability of anti-*Helicobacter pylori* treatment of peptic ulcers we are told: "why do you want to add an anti-ulcer procedure? Close the perforation and give a course of anti-Helicobacter antibiotics – the ulcer will be cured to never recur. This may be true, but in patients acutely operated for a perforated ulcer we do not know whether Helicobacter is or is not involved. Furthermore, particularly those patients who are susceptible to perforation also suffer from substandard access to medical care and reduced compliance, both adversely affecting successful medical anti-ulcer therapies. Consequently, if the operation for a perforated ulcer can kill two birds using one bullet – why not do it?

In What Patients Is a Definitive Procedure Safe?

Surely you do not want to embark on a lengthy definitive procedure in a critically ill and septic patient. Over the years we encountered surgeons who omitted a definitive procedure because of "severe contamination", often quoting a myth that vagotomy in a perforated patient may "spread the infection into the mediastinum". The Hong Kong group showed that when the following three factors are present an anti-ulcer procedure can be safely performed: blood pressure>90 mmHg, operation within 48 hours of perforation, lack of associated medical illnesses. We found the APACHE II scoring system (chapter 5) useful in this situation as patients with perforated ulcers with scores less than 11 can tolerate a definitive procedure of any magnitude. Conversely, in patients with higher APACHE II scores the simplest operation should be performed.

Operative Treatment; Simple Closure

Classically, simple closure of the ulcer is best achieved by an omental Graham's patch also called *omentopexy*. A few "through all layers" interrupted sutures are placed through both edges of the perforation and are left untied; a pedicle of the greater omentum is created and flipped over the perforation; the sutures are then gently tied over the omentum in order not to strangulate it. Occasionally surgeons misunderstand this operation; they initially suture – close the perforation, covering the suture line with the omentum. However, the approximation of the edematous, friable edges of perforation can be troublesome. In all cases of postoperative duodenal fistula witnessed by us the simple suture – closure of perforated DU was the causative mechanism. *Remember, you do not stitch the perforation but plug it with a viable omentum.*

Omentopexy can be easily performed for most perforated DU's. Rarely, a giant perforated DU creates a huge anterior bulbar – pyloric defect, which is not amenable to safe closure – mandating a partial gastrectomy.

Perforated GU's are usually larger than the duodenal ones. For those positioned on the greater curvature of the stomach, a wedge resection of the ulcer, hand sutured or stapled, may be easier and safer than omentopexy. For chronic and large lesser curvature ulcers, omentopexy is notoriously difficult and unsafe; partial gastrectomy may serve the patient better.

Operative Treatment; Definitive Procedure

Ideally, in emergency you should choose the anti-ulcer procedure with which you are most familiar in the elective situation. The problem is, however, that today you and other young surgeons are deprived of experience with elective anti-ulcer operations. Based on our philosophy to avoid, if possible, a gastric resection for a benign process, and on results of elective ulcer operations, we recommend an operative policy which

Table 13.1. Selection of procedures in perforated ulcers

| Ulcer type | Text book options | | We recommend | |
	Good risk	Poor risk	Good risk	Poor risk
Duodenal	omentopexy +/-TV+D or HSV or TV+A	omentopexy	omentopexy plus HSV	omentopexy
Prepyloric	omentopexy +/-TV+D or TV+A	omentopexy	omentopexy plus HSV+D	omentopexy
Gastric	omentopexy or wedge excision or partial gastrectomy	omentopexy or partial gastrectomy	omentopexy plus HSV+D or partial gastrectomy	omentopexy or partial gastrectomy

TV+D = trancal vagotomy and drainage procedure
HSV = highly selective vagotomy
TV+A = trancal vagotomy and antrectomy

tailors the definitive procedure to the specific ulcer (table 13.1). Whatever
you do – remember – if your patient is "sick" and you are not a skilled
gastroduodenal surgeon – forget about the definitive procedure – patch
the hole and get out!

Special Problems

"Kissing" Ulcers

Any evidence of a preceding or co-existing UGI hemorrhage (e.g. finding
of "coffee ground" or fresh blood in the NG tube or at the perforation
site or peritoneal cavity) suggests the presence of "kissing" ulcers: the
anterior perforated, the posterior bleeding. Simple closure of the former,
without hemostasis for the latter, could lead to a severe postoperative
hemorrhage. In such circumstances enlarge the duodenal perforation into a duodenotomy and explore the inside of the duodenum. If posterior
ulcer is found suture-transfix it's base as described in chapter 12.

Laparoscopic Management of Perforated Ulcers

Omentopexy and peritoneal toilet can be executed laparoscopically
(chapter 41) A large experience has been accumulated in the treatment
of perforated DU's with conflicting results. We suggest that laparoscopic
procedure is a reasonable option in stable and well-resuscitated patients
and when the perforation can be promptly and securely closed. Conversely, a prolonged pneumoperitoneum will be poorly tolerated in the
high risk or severely septic patients. The addition of a laparoscopic anti-
ulcer procedure could lengthen the operation beyond what is reasonable
in an emergency situation.

104   ## Non-Operative Management of Perforated Ulcers

Non-operative approach consisting of nil per mouth, nasogastric suction, systemic antibiotics, and acid secretion inhibitors, has been proven effective by a few enthusiastic groups. The sine qua non-for success is the spontaneous sealing of the perforation by the omentum or other adjacent structures; if this occurs non-operative approach would be successful in the majority of cases.

Non-operative treatment may be of particular value for two types of patients: the 'late presenter' and the "extremely sick". The former presents to you a day or more after the perforation occurred, with an already improving clinical picture and minimal abdominal findings. This, together with a radiographic evidence of free air, hints to a localized and spontaneously sealed perforation. Non-operative treatment, following a gastrografin UGI study to document that the perforation is sealed, should be successful in most instances. Other candidates for conservative therapy are those in whom the risk of any operation could be prohibitive, such as the early post massive MI patient, the COPD grade IV, or the patient with an APACHE II score over 25. Also in this group, however, conservative treatment may be successful only if the perforation is sealed and radiographically proven to be so. When sealing did not occur, in desperate situations we have successfully carried out omentopexy under local anesthesia.

Antibiotics

As soon as the diagnosis of perforation is made, and the patient is "booked" for a laparotomy, administer a dose of wide spectrum antibiotics. The vast majority of patients present for treatment within 12 hours of perforation and suffer, therefore, from peritoneal *contamination* rather than *infection*. In many of them, in fact, the peritonitis is chemical and does not contain any microorganisms. Antibiotics in this group will

serve for prophylaxis. Postoperative therapeutic antibiotics are not needed   105
in these patients. Those who present later than 12 hours may suffer from
intra-abdominal infection; here antibiotics should be continued in the
post-operative phase (chapter 32). The antibiotics given, either in a
form of "mono" or combination therapy, should "cover", empirically,
gram-negative and anaerobes. Routine culturing of the peritoneal fluid
in perforated patients is not indicated (chapters 6, 10 & 32). Those who
practice it (unnecessarily, we believe) often grow *Candida* species which
represents a contaminant and does not need specific therapy.

Conclusions

Patch perforated ulcer if you can, if you cannot, then you must resect.
Consider adding a definitive anti-ulcer procedure on a selective basis,
and do not forget that non-operative approach is possible and indicated
in selective patients.

14 Acute Pancreatitis

*Everything in surgery is complicated until one learns to do it well,
then it is easy*
(Robert E. Condon)

Most attacks of acute pancreatitis (AP) are mild to moderate and resolve
spontaneously. This chapter concentrates on the complications of AP,
which may require emergency abdominal surgery.

Classification

Emergency surgery is usually reserved for the treatment of the uncommon
necrotic and infective complications of severe AP. The latter include a
large spectrum of conditions, which may develop following an attack of
severe AP of any etiology:
- Pancreatic & peri-pancreatic necrosis
- Infected pancreatic & peri-pancreatic necrosis (IPN)
- Pancreatic abscess
- Pseudocyst
- Infected pseudocyst

Natural History

Recognize that an uncomplicated attack of AP is *"a one week disease"*.
Failure to recover and persistence of local and systemic signs of pancreatic
inflammation beyond the 7th day, hints that a complication may loom at
the background. You'll best understand this complicated disease, and
develop a rational clinical approach to treat it, when considering it week
by week – as it evolves (Figure 14.1).

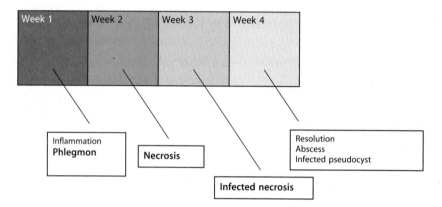

Fig 14.1. Natural history of complicated acute pancreatitis

First Week: Inflammation

This is the phase of acute inflammation resulting in an inflammatory mass, which consist of the pancreas and adjacent structures – "pancreatic phlegmon". Pro-inflammatory mediators (e.g. cytokines) are present in the dark brown – hemorrhagic – exudate of severe AP, producing the local and systemic clinical picture of inflammation. The systemic repercussions of AP (e.g. respiratory or renal failure) depend on the intensity of the process and the quantity of mediators entering the retroperitoneum, the peritoneal cavity and the circulation.

Second Week: Necrosis

This is the phase of necrosis, which starts towards the end of the first week. The necrotizing process may involve the pancreas and its surroundings; its retroperitoneal spread hastened by activated proteolytic pancreatic enzymes. The severity of disease and prognosis depend on

the quantity and extent of necrotic tissue (sometimes involving the 109
whole retroperitoneum) and whether a secondary infection supervenes.
Pooling of the exudate in the lesser sac and beyond forms the so-called
acute peri-pancreatic fluid collections, which may resolve spontaneously,
or develop an inflammatory wall to become a *pancreatic pseudocyst*.

Third Week: Infection

This is the phase of infection. The diagnostic modalities described below
may point to infection of the necrosed tissue already in the middle of
the second week, but its peak incidence is the third week. The causative
organisms probably originate from the nearby colon by translocation.
The resulting infection of necrotic tissue produces *infected pancreatic
and/or peri-pancreatic necrosis*, whereas secondary infection of a
pseudocyst results in an *infected pseudocyst* (a rarer and more benign
process). The combined effects of necrosis and infection give rise to the
clinical scenario at this stage, both associated with local and systemic
inflammatory syndromes. IPN may occasionally produce a relatively
mild systemic illness, while widespread sterile necrosis may cause the
patient's demise, the outcome depending probably on the intensity of the
inflammatory response in the individual patient.

Fourth Week and Beyond

Patients with non-infected pancreatic and/or peri-pancreatic necrosis,
whose hitherto relatively benign clinical course did not mandate an
operation, enter this "late" phase. We do not know what is the quantity of
necrotic pancreatic parenchyma, which can resolve spontaneously. We
know, however, that even large necrotic zones may be reabsorbed and
undergo secondary infection, to present weeks later as a *pancreatic abscess*.
This is an infective localized process developing after the resolution of
the acute pancreatic inflammatory process. Therefore, the presentation,

110   management and prognosis of pancreatic abscess differ drastically with that of IPN. Pseudocysts may also develop at this stage and become infected.

Estimation of the Severity of Illness

Severe AP will eventually declare itself by failing to resolve or its dramatic systemic effects. It is important for you to recognize early that the attack is severe in order to optimize the patient care, prevent infective complications, and evaluate the prognosis.

Levels of specific pancreatic enzymes or acute phase reactants were reported to correlate with the severity of disease and outcome but it is unlikely that one or two biochemical tests would suffice. Dark-brown or murky peritoneal fluid is diagnostic of necrotizing-hemorrhagic pancreatitis (i.e. severe AP). This requires, however, peritoneal aspiration which represents an invasive procedure and not accepted as a routine in the early phase of AP.

A number of scoring systems were developed to estimate the severity of AP. Most are based on clinical and laboratory variables which reflect the intensity of the inflammatory process. Imrie's method is popular in the UK, whereas any medical student in the world knows about Ranson's criteria. The APACHE II scoring system is useful to measure the severity of *any acute disease*, and has been shown to better prognosticate the outcome of AP than any other system. We advise you to use this uniform and user-friendly scoring system (chapter 5). *A patient with an APACHE II score of more than 8 has a severe AP.*

Contrast-enhanced dynamic computed tomography has been reported to be useful in diagnosing AP and grading its severity. The clinical diagnosis of AP is, however, straightforward and scoring can assess the severity of disease better. Moreover, the contrast-enhanced CT examination has been implicated in the aggravation of the microvascular damage in the pancreatic parenchyma. In addition, CT findings during

the first week of AP very rarely will influence management decisions.
We suggest that you avoid CT scanning the AP patient in the early phase
of the disease and reserve this examination for patients in whom the
diagnosis of AP is uncertain. Ultrasound should, however, be performed
to confirm or exclude cholelithiasis.

Diagnostic & Therapeutic Approach

The optimal diagnostic and management pathways are still controversial.
It will be discussed in the order of its clinical occurrence – again – week
by week.

Inflammation-First Week

Generally, the approach to early severe AP is *conservative* and the treatment *supportive*. Since pro-inflammatory mediators cause the clinical
manifestations there were attempts to prevent or diminish such response
with *early pancreatectomy or peritoneal lavage*, respectively. Pancreatic
resection in early severe AP is associated with a horrendous mortality
rate and does not prevent the development of intra-abdominal infection.
Although continuous peritoneal lavage may improve systemic manifestations, if started early (within a day of two), it is clear that it does not
prevent the late major complications (and mortality) we are talking
about. "Filtration" of the blood off the noxious mediators liberated by AP
has been tried but remains experimental.

*It appears, therefore, that you should offer these patients nothing
more (and nothing less) than supportive care, preferably in the SICU.* You
should remember that severe AP represents a *major abdominal "chemical
burn"* with many liters of fluid sequestrated in the retroperitoneum and
peritoneal cavity. Optimal fluid balance and replacement are mandatory
to protect the kidneys and provide an adequate venous return to the

112   heart, which may be adversely affected by the pancreatitis-related myocardial depressing factor. Overhydration, on the other hand, should be
prevented especially in the presence of an associated ARDS. The swollen
pancreas, together with the edematous, SIRS-affected viscera, may easily
produce intra-abdominal hypertension. You won't know about it unless
you measure the intra-abdominal pressure. When abdominal compartment
syndrome complicates severe AP, the abdomen should be decompressed
(chapter 28).

We have always been told that "resting the pancreas" by gastric
decompression and nil per mouth regimen is beneficial. This remains
unproven. Gastric decompression with a nasogastric tube should be
employed only in the presence of gastric ileus or outlet obstruction due
to the swollen pancreas. Classically, the parenteral route was used for
nutritional support but recent evidence suggests that enteral nutrition
via a transduodenal tube is well tolerated and results in less local and
systemic complications (chapter 31).

Evidence suggests that intravenous antibiotics are to be started in
any AP patient assessed as "severe". This serves to prevent superinfection
of the necrotic tissue, thus reducing the incidence of IPN. *Imipenem*, a
wide spectrum agent, which achieves high levels within the pancreatic
parenchyma appears to be the drug of choice. Some authorities recommend
the addition of an anti-fungal (e.g. fluconazole) agent to prevent fungal
superinfection of the necrotic pancreas.

As already mentioned, there is no indication at this stage to obtain
a CT scan unless you are insecure about your diagnosis. Laparotomy is
almost contra-indicated during early AP and should be allowed only in
cases where a life-threatening surgical catastrophe cannot be otherwise
excluded. Another rare indication for a laparotomy at this phase is to
decompress an *abdominal compartment syndrome* as mentioned above.
Indeed, *exploratory laparotomy in AP is not innocuous*; in fact, it adversely
affects the natural history of the disease by increasing the incidence of
infective complications.

Endoscopic sphincterotomy is the only invasive therapeutic modality   113
that could be considered – early during the first week in the course of severe
biliary AP, especially if features of ascending cholangitis are present.

Your dedicated supportive care will result in the survival of most
of these patients – when their disease process enters the second week.

Necrosis-Second Week

Pancreatic necrosis develops in one fifth of patients suffering of AP who
have more than 3 Ranson's criteria or an APACHE II score higher than 8.
Dynamic, contrast-enhanced CT is the best way to diagnose necrosis and
should be obtained in patients who are not improving towards the end
of the first week. CT examination at this stage serves also as a "base-line"
for subsequent imaging. Pancreatic parenchyma that does not pick up
contrast is considered necrotic; the volume of necrosis is then estimated
relative to the well-perfused area.

Once pancreatic necrosis is diagnosed, you must answer two
questions:
- *Is the process infected (i.e. IPN)?*
- *Is an operation indicated, and if so, which?*

The probability of infection is very low at the beginning of the second
week but it gradually increases, reaching its peak in the third week. Because
it is impossible to clinically distinguish between sterile and infected
necrosis, additional diagnostic modalities are necessary. Gas bubbles in
the region of the pancreas are observed on plain radiographs or CT in a
third of infected cases, and are pathognomonic. If no air bubbles are seen
then fine needle CT-guided aspiration of necrotic tissue for Gram stain
and culture is necessary. *Bacterial infection of pancreatic or peri-pancreatic*
necrosis is lethal if left untreated and therefore represent an absolute
indication for operation.

How to treat non-infected necrosis? This is controversial. On one hand, massive sterile necrosis is responsible for severe morbidity and even death; furthermore, necrosis may lead to IPN. On the other hand, we know that sterile necrosis may resolve spontaneously. It is not clear, however, whether or not very large segments (more than a half) of the pancreatic parenchyma may respond to conservative therapy. These uncertainties led to different approaches. Partial pancreatic resections to eradicate the involved areas have been performed, at the price of excessive morbidity and mortality. Often, normal parenchyma is excised as both radiologists and surgeons tend to overestimate the extent of necrosis. At the other side of spectrum, there are those who would persist with conservative treatment for as long as possible, waiting for the demarcation of necrotic tissue which would facilitate the eventual operation. We suggest an intermediate approach, mandating surgery in the presence of clear evidence of infection or deterioration of the "patient on maximal supportive treatment", even in the absence of documented lobal infection. A "stable" patient with sterile necrosis should be subjected to serial CT examinations and fine needle aspirations. Operation becomes necessary in the third or fourth week if either infection is uncovered or the patient fails to recover.

Infection (or Resolution), Pseudocyst – Third Week

During this phase most patients with IPN undergo an operation, while those with sterile necrosis begin to recover. The resolution of necrosis may result in the formation of a pseudocyst diagnosed on CT or ultrasonography. If signs of infection are present a diagnostic needle aspiration should be carried out. *The treatment of choice of an infected pseudocyst is percutaneous drainage.*

Pancreatic Abscess-Fourth Week and Beyond 115

In some other cases of pancreatic necrosis treated non-operatively, resolution does not occur. Instead, a collection of pus – *pancreatic abscess* –
forms in the retroperitoneum. Generally, these patients are less severely
sick than those with IPN. Nevertheless, drainage by one or other means
is indicated.

Operative Approach

Percutaneous (PC) Drainage

Successful CT or ultrasound-guided PC drainage of isolated intra-abdominal
abscesses (chapter 35) has prompted attempts at a similar approach in
AP-related collections. Clearly, PC drains are able to remove exudate and
thin pus but inadequate to evacuate the thick "junk" typical of IPN.
Thus, PC drainage may be successful in the treatment of isolated early
peri-pancreatic fluid collections, infected and non- infected pseudocysts
or the late-occurring isolated pancreatic abscess. *When your patient fails
to improve within 24–48 hours of PC drainage consider surgery. PC drainage
is doomed to fail when infected pancreatic necrosis is present; this always
requires an operation.*

The Operation

The surgical approach to infected or non-infected pancreatic necrosis is
essentially the same, evolving around the removal of necrotic tissue.
(It is hoped that you won't have too many opportunities to operate on
sterile necrosis). The key issues are:
- *Timing* (early versus late) as discussed above.
- *Approach* (trans-peritoneal versus retroperitoneal)

116

- *Technique* (pancreatic resection versus removal of necrotic tissue – necrosectomy)
- *Management of wound* (closure of the abdomen versus open management – laparostomy)
- *Postoperative management* (with or without continuous irrigation of the pancreatic bed)
- *Re-operations* ("Planned" versus "on-demand")

You can approach the site of necrosis from the front, trans-peritoneally, or extra-peritoneally, via a flank incision. The latter prevents contamination of the peritoneal cavity and could decrease the incidence of wound complications. This "blind" technique is associated however with a higher risk of injury to the transverse colon and retroperitoneal hemorrhage. In addition, it makes proper exploration and necrosectomy difficult. We prefer therefore a trans-peritoneal approach through a long transverse incision (Chevron) which offers generous exposure of the entire abdomen. A midline incision offers adequate exposure but interferes with the small bowel in cases where planned re-operations or laparostomy are subsequently necessary (chapter 37). The extra-peritoneal routes are valuable in rare instances when the process is localized at the pancreatic tail, on the left side, or its head, on the right. It is more often used to evacuate localized "sequesters" of necrotic fat during subsequent re-operations.

Your main objectives at operation are:

- To evacuate the necrotic and infected material
- To drain the toxic products of the process
- To prevent re-accumulation of these products
- To avoid injury to adjacent visceral and vascular structures

We should emphasize that pancreatic necrosis/infection is drastically different from other surgical infections you are called to treat, as the pancreatic process tends to progress despite an apparently adequate initial debridement and drainage.

The three main operative approaches practiced today are:

- Debridement, wide drainage and abdominal closure. Further procedures are carried out on "on demand".
- As above plus continuous, local irrigation of the lesser sac (for a few weeks!) With re-operations performed "on demand".
- The "aggressive" method, which includes leaving the abdomen open (laparostomy) and planned re-laparotomies to repeatedly debride the necrotizing process until it is completely eradicated (chapter 37). Another theoretical advantage of this method is that it prevents the development of the *abdominal compartment syndrome* due to increased intra-abdominal pressure, which results from the swelling of the pancreas, accumulation of necrotic material and fluid, and visceral edema.

What is the "best" approach? It appears that significantly lower mortality rates are achieved with the last two methods. The third method is associated with higher rate of "mechanical re-operative" complications including hemorrhage, fistulaization of the transverse colon and abdominal wall defects. *It is clear that the mainstay of therapy is the complete evacuation of IPN and that too conservative approach in the face of a diffuse process is the chief cause of mortality.*

Each of the three methods may succeed in a certain patient and should be used selectively depending on the extent of IPN and severity of the illness in the individual patient. The first approach may suffice in a patient with a localized process and small quantity of necrosis. The second technique may be advantageous when a more extensive process is limited to the lesser sac. Extensive IPN, however, requires the most aggressive treatment

118   as represented by the third method, which is life saving when the process
extends diffusely in the retroperitoneum

Practical Operative Points

When operating on pancreatic necrosis or IPN you must understand
that it is often impossible to be performing a definitive debridement.
Leave the rest for tomorrow (e.g. re-operation). Over-enthusiastic debridement will debride the bowel (which will leak) or adjacent vessels
(which will bleed). Follow the necrotizing process down the retroperitoneum; it may extend behind the left and right colon into the pelvis. Only
the soft necrotic black gray Camembert cheese-like material should be
necrosectomized. Using your fingers or a blunt sponge forceps to pick up
the material will avoid the hard – non-necrotic pancreas and other
structures.

Enter the lesser sac from whatever direction it is easier, but expose
it completely. *Try not to add harm.* This is easier said than done while
burrowing within inflamed and friable tissues. Safeguard the vessels in
the transverse mesocolon; these are commonly injured during trans-me-
socolon entry into the lesser sac or by drains placed through this route.
It is tempting to remove the spleen, which may take part in an inflammatory mass in the pancreatic tail. This is not necessary; try to not injure the spleen during re-operations. The adherent duodenum and loops
of small bowel are frequently injured during re-operations; this together
with the corrosive action of activated pancreatic enzymes causes intestinal leaks. Be extremely gentle with the bowel and avoid rigid drains near
the duodenum for they will erode. Often after necrosectomy there is diffuse ooze from the resulting cavity. Pack it! Try not to place packs directly on exposed veins- they will erode and bleed! Safeguard the omentum
and place it between the packs and exposed vessels. More on the con-
duction of laparostomy see in chapter 37.

Conclusions

The proper management of severe acute pancreatitis requires that you understand its natural history and be armed with lot of patience. During the early phases of the disease *our patience will achieve more than our force" (Edmund Burke)*; later on, when called to operate on necrotic and infected complications, remember that ...

"patience and diligence, like faith, remove mountains"
(William Penn).

15 Acute Cholecystitis

When the gallbladder is "diffuclt" –
go fundus down and stay near the wall.

Acute cholecystitis (AC) is either *calculous* or, less commonly, *acalculous.*
Since the clinical picture of these two entities differs they are discussed
separately.

Calculous Acute Cholecystitis

Acute cholecystitis is initiated by a gallstone, which obstructs the gallbladder's
outlet. It's spontaneous dislodgment results in the so called *biliary colic*
while persisting impaction of the stone produces gallbladder distention
and inflammation, namely *AC*. The latter is chemical initially but gradually,
as gut bacteria invade the inflamed organ, infection supervenes. The combination of distention, ischemia, and infection may result in a gallbladder
empyema, necrosis, perforation, peri-cholecystic abscess or bile-peritonitis.
You must have heard or read numerous times about the classical symptoms and signs of AC. Let us concentrate therefore only on problem areas.

How to differentiate between biliary colic and AC? Time is the best
arbitrator as the pain and RUQ symptoms of biliary colic are self limited,
disappearing within a few hours. Conversely, in AC, the symptoms and
signs persist. Furthermore, AC is accompanied by local (e.g. local
peritonitis or tender mass) and systemic (e.g. fever, leukocytosis) evidence
of inflammation, while biliary colic is not.

The clinical picture that you know so well (we do not need to
mention Murphy's sign again) is very suggestive. Laboratory findings of
leukocytosis and elevation of bilirubin and/or liver enzymes may back
it. But note that lack of a few or more features of inflammation/infection
does not rule out AC – as is true also for acute appendicitis.

122   Luckily, you can (and should) confirm your diagnosis of AC with the *ultrasound* or *radionuclide HIDA scan*, which are readily available. Which of the two should you ask for first depends on its availability, and the expertise in your hospital. We prefer the ultrasound as it may also provide "side information" concerning the liver, bile ducts, pancreas, kidney and peritoneal fluid, thus suggesting alternative diagnoses. The *ultrasonographic findings in AC* include a distended, stone or sludge-containing gallbladder, thickened wall, mucosal separation, peri-chole-cystic fluid collection or intramural air. Not all of these findings are necessary to make a diagnosis. Positive radionuclide scan in AC means the non-filling of the gallbladder. The specificity of the test is increased (i.e. less false positive) if morphine is administered, causing spasm of the sphincter of Oddi and reflux of isotope into the cystic duct. There are other causes of non-filling of the gallbladder (e.g. mucocele) but *a negative scan-isotope entering the gallbladder – excludes AC.*

Associated Jaundice

Mild to moderate elevation of bilirubin and hepatic enzymes is a relatively common feature of AC, caused by reactive inflammation of the hepatic pedicle and liver parenchyma. Thus, in the absence of clinical and ultra-sonographic features of ascending cholangitis and bile duct stones, respectively, you should not attribute the jaundice to choledocholithiasis (chapter 16).

Associated Hyperamylesemia

Similarly, not in every AC patient in whom serum amylase is elevated should acute biliary pancreatitis be diagnosed. Commonly, the hyper-amylesemia is produced by AC with no signs of acute pancreatitis detected at operation.

Management

Conservative Management

The natural history of AC is such that in more than two-thirds of patients treated conservatively the increased intra-gallbladder pressure results in the dislodgment of the obstructing stone and resolution of the process. Conservative therapy, which should be started in all AC patients after the establishment of diagnosis, includes: nil per mouth (nasogastric tube only if the patient is vomiting), analgesia (use a non-opioid if you believe in the hypothetical importance of not to constrict the sphincter of Oddi), and antibiotics (active against enteric gram-negative bacteria).

In the "old days" patients were discharged home after responding to a few days of conservative treatment to return for a *delayed,"interval",* *cholecystectomy* a few weeks later. This approach has been discontinued because of unpredictable failure to respond and recurrences of AC prior to the planned operation. Today, we reserve *delayed cholecystectomy* to patients who are medically unfit to undergo an operation at this stage, provided they responded to conservative management.

Surgical Management

Cholecystectomy is the optimal procedure, which eradicates the inflammation/infection and prevents its recurrence. Based on your clinical impression it will be performed either as an "emergency" or "early".

Emergency Cholecystectomy
An immediate, emergency procedure should be performed following resuscitation in patients with clinical evidence of *diffuse peritonitis ,* *systemic toxicity, a palpable inflammatory mass in the right upper quadrant* or *presence of gas within the gallbladder wall* – features suggesting perforation, necrosis or empyema of the gallbladder. Some surgeons may

124   attempt a trial laparoscopic cholecystectomy (LC) in this situation, converting to "open" in the presence of technical difficulties. We, however, do not support peritoneal insufflation in the critically ill patient and would ovoid laparoscopic dissection of the necrotic, perforated and difficult to grasp gallbladder. Emergency cholecystectomy for complicated AC should be "open" as described below.

Early Cholecystectomy

Patients in whom emergency cholecystectomy is not clinically indicated should undergo an early cholecystectomy. *But what is "early"?* For some it means that you do not need to rush to the OR in the middle of the night but operate during day-hours, under favorable "elective" conditions. For others it means to operate on the "first elective list". Depending on surgeons' schedule and the availability of the OR, patients are often left "to cool down" for days awaiting their "semi-elective" cholecystectomy, which is often performed at the end of the elective lists. Occasionally, waiting periods as short as 48 hours resulted in the deterioration of the patient.

The clinical appraisal of the severity of AC is notoriously unreliable: patients with gallbladder empyema or necrosis may be initially clinically silent only to suddenly deteriorate while those with impressive RUQ findings may harbor just a simple AC. A mandatory operation within 24 hours will prevent any pitfalls arising from a delay to operate. Furthermore, the operative dissection (laparoscopic or open) is easier and less "bloody" during the early phase of inflammation, with tissue plans becoming progressively more "difficult" as the process progresses. *Thus, our definition of early cholecystectomy is an operation within 24 hours of admission.*

Note: there is a subgroup of patients who will benefit from a waiting period, in order to better prepare them for surgery. For example, decompensated cardiac failure should be treated and coagulation disturbances corrected. Do not 'jump' immediately with the knife on unprepared patients.

The High Risk Patient
Who Needs an Emergency Procedure

With today's advanced anesthetic techniques and ICU support it is rare to encounter a patient who "cannot be subjected to an emergency procedure under GA". But what to do with the occasional extremely sick patent who is even "not fit for a hair cut under local" – as they used to say? The options are a *tube cholecystostomy* under local anesthesia; either ultra-sound guided, per cutaneous-transhepatic, by the radiologist or an operative cholecystostomy -performed by you. Failure of the patient to improve within 24 hours, particularly after the percutaneous procedure, should suggest the presence of undrained pus or necrotic gallbladder wall, *and the need to operate.*

Acute Cholecystitis in Cirrhotic Patients

An emergency cholecystectomy in cirrhotic – portal hypertension – patients not uncommonly culminates into a *bloody disaster* due to an intra- or postoperative hemorrhage from the congested gallbladder's hepatic bed or large venous collaterals at the duodenohepatic ligament. Although conventional laparoscopic cholecystectomy has been judged as safe in selected "Child A" portal hypertension patients, we believe that the secret here is to stay away from trouble, namely not to dissect near engorged and rigid hepatic parenchyma and the excessively vascular triangle of Callot. Subtotal or partial cholecystectomy is the procedure of choice in this situation – as discussed below.

Technical Points

Cholecystectomy

As aforementioned, many "*emergency*" procedures will be "open" unless you like to play around with the laparoscope in desperately ill patients. In "*early*" cholecystectomy you may start laparoscopically, accepting a need to convert to "open" in up to one third of the patients. It is important not to be carried away, persisting with laparoscopic dissection in face of hostile anatomy. A practical rule of thumb is to convert to laparotomy if after 45–60 minutes of laparoscopy you feel like you are "proceeding nowhere".

There is no need to further educate you on the topic of laparoscopic cholecystectomy. You may need, however, some advice on the open procedure, which is becoming rare in your practice but being reserved to the "difficult" cases, ever more challenging.

The *routine*, "maxi", full-size gallbladder abdominal incision belongs to history. In the acute situation start with a "midi"-5 to 10 cm' transverse RUQ incision, extending "piecemeal" as necessary. The wise-man's rule is: "*go fundus down and stay near the gallbladder*". After needle – decompressing (connect a wide-bore needle to the suction) of the distended gallbladder, hold the fundus up with an instrument and dissect down towards the cystic duct and artery which are the last attachments to be secured and divided. Observing this rule it is virtually impossible to damage anything significant such as the bile duct.

Subtotal (Partial) Cholecystectomy

This is the procedure to use, in order to avoid misery, in problematic situations such as difficult to dissect triangle of Callot, portal hypertension, or coagulopathy. The gallbladder is resected starting at the fundus; the posterior wall (or what has remained of it when a necrotizing attack has occurred) is left attached to the hepatic bed and its rim is oversewn for

hemostasis with a running suture. At the level of the Hartmann pouch,
the cystic duct opening is identified from within. The accurate placement
of a purse-string suture around this opening as described by others is
not satisfactory, as the suture tends to tear out in the inflamed and friable
tissues. Best is to leave a 1 cm rim of the Hartmann pouch tissue and
suture-buttress it over the opening of the cystic duct. When no healthy
gallbladder wall remains to close the cystic duct, it is absolutely safe just
to leave a suction drain and bail out. In the absence of distal common
bile duct obstruction you won't see even a drop of bile in the drain because
in such cases the cystic duct is obstructed due the inflammatory process.
The exposed and often necrotic mucosa of the posterior gallbladder wall
is destroyed with diathermy and the omentum is brought into the area.
In this operation the structures in the Callot's triangle are not dissected
out and bleeding from the hepatic bed is avoided; it is a fast and safe
procedure having the advantages of both cholecystectomy and cholecystostomy.

Cholecystostomy

In our hands, subtotal cholecystectomy has almost replaced "open" tube
cholecystostomy for the "difficult" gallbladder. This procedure is indicated
in the very rare patient who *must* be done under local anesthesia and
when percutaneous cholecystostomy is not available or successful. After
the infiltration of local anesthesia place a "mini" incision over the point
of maximum tenderness or the palpable GB mass. You can mark the
position of the fundus on the skin at the pre-operative ultrasound as it is
rather unpleasant for both you and the patient to enter the abdomen,
under local anesthesia, and find that the gallbladder is faraway. The visualization of gallbladder wall necrosis at this stage mandates a subtotal
cholecystectomy; otherwise open the fundus and remove all stones from
the gallbladder and its' Hartmann's pouch. For improved inspection of
the gallbladder's lumen, and complete extraction of stones and sludge,

128   a sterile proctoscope may be useful. Thereafter, insert into the fundus a tube of your choice (we prefer a large Foley), securing it in place with a purse-string suture. Fix the fundus to the cholecystostomy site at the abdominal wall, as you would do with a gastrostomy. A tube cholangiogram performed a week after the operation will tell you whether the cystic duct and bile ducts are patent; if so the tube can be safely removed. Whether an interval cholecystectomy is subsequently indicated is controversial.

Choledocholithiasis Associated With Acute Cholecystitis

About a tenth of patients who suffer from AC have also stones in their bile ducts. Remember, however, that AC may produce jaundice and liver enzyme disturbances in the absence of any ductal pathology. AC is very rarely associated with active complications of choledocholithiasis. Thus, the "combinations" of AC with acute pancreatitis, ascending cholangitis, or *obstructive* jaundice are uncommon. The emphasis, therefore, should be on the treatment of AC, which represent the life-threatening condition; ductal stones, if present, are of secondary importance – at this stage.

Our management of patients with diagnosed AC with suspected choledocholithiasis would consist of a cholecystectomy (as outlined above) combined with intra-operative cholangiogram. Should the latter be positive we would proceed with a common bile duct exploration, converting to an open procedure if the initial approach was laparoscopic. Of course, if you are skilled in laparoscopic trans-cystic common bile duct exploration-have go at it. In the critically ill patient with or without gallbladder empyema or perforation we would even "waive" the cholangiogram, leaving the symptomatic ductal stones to endoscopic retrieval after the life-saving cholecystectomy or cholecystostomy.

Acalculous Cholecystitis   129

It is another common sequel to the disturbed micro-circulation in the critically-ill patients. Although of *multifactorial etiology* (e.g. prolonged fasting, TPN administration, etc) the common pathogenic pathway is probably gallbladder ischemia, mucosal injury and secondary bacterial invasion. Acalculous cholecystitis is a *life-threatening condition* developing during a serious illness such as following major surgery or severe injury. Stones may occasionally be present in the acutely inflamed gallbladders under these circumstances but are probably etiologically irrelevant.

Clinical diagnosis is extremely difficult in the critically ill or traumatized patient. Abdominal complaints and the background disease mask signs. Fever, jaundice, leukocytosis and disturbed liver function tests are commonly present but are entirely nonspecific. The early diagnosis requires a high index of suspicion on your side: *suspect & exclude cholecystitis as the cause of an otherwise unexplained "septic state" or SIRS.*

Ultrasonography performed at the bedside is the diagnostic modality of choice. Gallbladder-*wall thickness* (>3.0–3.5 mm), *intramural gas*, the *"halo" sign* and *pericholecystic fluid*, are very suggestive. Similar findings on *CT*-examination would confirm the diagnosis. False-positive and negative studies have been reported with both imaging modalities. *Hepatobiliary radio-isotope* scanning is associated with a high incidence of false-positive studies. However, *filling of the gallbladder with the radio-isotope (morphine assisted, if necessary) excludes cholecystitis.* Highly suggestive clinical scenario and diagnostic uncertainty is an indication for abdominal exploration.

Bedside laparoscopy (under local anesthesia) offers excellent direct view of the gallbladder to confirm or exclude the diagnosis. *Note:* Insufflation pressure during laparoscopy should be kept under 10 mmHg in order not to upset the flimsy cardio-respiratory balance and hemodynamics in such patients

Management should be promptly instituted as acalculous cholecystitis progresses rapidly to necrosis and perforation. *Select* the best treatment modality based on the condition of your patient and the expertise available in your hospital. In patients stable enough to undergo general anesthesia *cholecystectomy* is indicated. When coagulopathy, portal hypertension or severe inflammatory obliteration of the triangle of Callot are present, *subtotal cholecystectomy* appears to be safer. *Laparoscopic cholecystectomy* may be performed in well-selected and stable patients.

"Open" tube cholecystostomy under local anesthesia may be indicated in the moribund patient when expertise for *percutaneous, transhepatic cholecystostomy* is not locally available. The latter is probably the procedure of choice in the severely ill patient when diagnostic certainty is strong.

Remember: Many of these patients will have a totally necrotic or perforated gallbladder. In these, cholecystostomy may not suffice. *Percutaneous cholecystostomy* is a *blind* procedure; when rapid resolution of 'sepsis' does not follow suspect local residuals of pus or necrosis, or an alternative intra-abdominal or systemic diagnosis.

Antibiotics in Acute Cholecystitis

Although routinely administered the role of antibiotics is only adjunctive to the operative treatment as outlined above. In its early phase AC represent a sterile inflammation while later on in most instances it represents a 'resectable infection'-(chapter 10) e.g. infection contained within the gallbladder which is to be removed. Therefore, cases with simple AC need only peri-operative antibiotic 'coverage', to be discontinued postoperatively. In gangrene or 'contained' empyema of the gallbladder we recommend a day or two of post-cholecystectomy antibiotic administration. In cases of perforation with a peri-cholecystic abscess or bile peritonitis we suggest that you administer the "maximal" postoperative course of 5 days (chapter 32).

16 Acute Cholangitis

That an emergency operation is very rarely indicated
in acute cholangitis does not mean that it is never indicated

What Is the Mechanism?

Acute ascending cholangitis is an infectious-inflammatory consequence
of biliary obstruction. Biliary stasis results in translocation of organisms
and a cascade of problems that can result in death if not treated appropriately. Cholangitis may arise in the liver or it may 'ascend' from an
obstruction arising in the extra-hepatic biliary tree. It is the latter which
we, as surgeons, most commonly have to treat. The two common causes
of extra-hepatic biliary obstruction are *common bile duct stones and*
pancreatic (or periampullary) carcinoma with the former much more
common than the latter. Less frequently, the distal common bile duct can
be 'cicatrized' as a result of chronic pancreatitis. Postoperative biliary
strictures are becoming rather common "thanks" to laparoscopic biliary
surgery with its inherent (increased) risk of bile duct injury. Typical of
cholangitis arising from choledocholithiasis is the prior history of
'fluctuant' jaundice. The patient may also admit to having had gallstones
diagnosed in the past or may have had a prior cholecystectomy.

What Are the Risks?

It is always a good idea to know who is likely to die from a disease and
why, before you decide how to proceed from the emergency room (ER),
through the hospital, and occasionally to the morgue! Like any acute
illness, age, associated cardio-respiratory compromise caused by the
current event, and the patient's prior medical problems, all contribute to

132 his/her risk of dying from acute cholangitis. It is always useful to run an APACHE II baseline in the ER and keep a mental note of the changes as you monitor your patient to ensure that your interventions or lack thereof, are not causing a rise in your patient's score (chapter 5). As a rule in this condition, the direct bilirubin decreases as the treatment takes effect.

How To Make the Diagnosis?

Charcot's Triad characterizes acute ascending cholangitis:
- Right upper quadrant pain
- Fever
- Jaundice

The fever and jaundice are easy to determine. It is our experience that residents miss the objective distinction between the clinical finding of a tender liver which is the cause of the RUQ pain in cholangitis and Murphy's Sign, which is a sign of gallbladder obstruction. *Murphy's Sign* is elicited by the presence of point tenderness in the region of the distended gallbladder fundus as it descends to the awaiting fingertips of the right hand on deep inspiration. The RUQ tenderness seen in acute cholangitis is objective percussion-tenderness elicited along the width of the liver, especially in the epigastrium where the left lobe is not shielded by the costal margin. In addition, there is usually a varying degree of liver swelling which makes this sign easier to elicit. If correctly identified in the ER 'cot-side', the treatment for cholangitis is begun before one sends the patient for the customary HIDA scan to rule out an obstructed gallbladder and which is absolutely unnecessary and misleading in patients with cholangitis. Indeed, it is also for this reason that we prefer RUQ ultrasonography as the initial investigation in all patients with suspected cholecystitis/biliary colic rather than the ubiquitous HIDA scan (chapter 15).

What Are Signs of Complications?

In the elderly patient, or when medical intervention is delayed, the syndrome can progress to include two further clinical features:

- Confusion (Do not assume that any elderly-confused patient in the ER has senile dementia, ask about the patient's baseline mental status).
- "Septic" shock

These two, when added to the *Charcot's Triad* become the *Reynold's Pentad*, which is associated with a four-fold mortality risk increase; consequently, clinical decision intervals must be hourly rather than q4h!

Special Investigations

Ascending cholangitis is diagnosed on the aforementioned clinical grounds. With early presentation, the jaundice may only be biochemical and must be substantiated by a liver panel. A typical panel has mildly elevated transaminases, variably elevated total bilirubin with a direct preponderance, and a disproportionately elevated alkaline phosphatase and glutamyl transferase. White cells are usually elevated with a "bandemia". Amylase may be mildly elevated (less than 5-fold elevation) but must not be confused with acute pancreatitis (chapter 14). Other laboratory data will be appropriate for the patient's degree of hydration and respiratory status, which can deteriorate rapidly if the patient presents late or the diagnosis is delayed.

The right upper quadrant sonogram is the best test to confirm the diagnosis. Invariable gallstones are seen in the gallbladder (unless the patient has had a prior cholecystectomy). Mild intra-hepatic ductal dilatation will be demonstrated and the common hepatic duct /common bile duct axis will be variably dilated above a normal level of 7 mm.

Rarely can the incriminating bile duct stone(s) be seen directly. Rather, their presence is inferred by the above associated findings. If gallstones are not seen in the gallbladder then the diagnosis of periampullary biliary obstruction must be suspected, justifying the performance of a thin slice pancreas protocol CT scan. This is usually requested after treatment is begun and during regular hours to prevent a substandard nocturnal study.

Treatment

Initial Management

Initial management comprises of appropriate empiric antibiotics with bowel rest and rehydration. Antibiotic selection is based upon the drug's ability to concentrate in the biliary system and its coverage against gram negative, gut-derived organisms (typically *E.coli* and *Klebsiella* sp). Most patients will defervesce within 24 hours on the above treatment. The remainder will have persistent fever and pain, and their bilirubin may rise, implying a persistent complete obstruction. It is at this time that urgent ERCP is indicated with sphincterotomy and stone extraction. It is the gastroenterologist's task to ensure biliary decompression at the first attempt. This does not mean complete duct clearance, as stones may be difficult to extract at one session. This may necessitate placement of a plastic biliary stent or nasobiliary tube. The latter's advantage is that it can be removed without re-endoscopy after cholecystectomy.

When or if ERCP fails in the critically ill cholangitis patient there is another non-operative alternative: ultrasound-guided percutaneous drainage of the obstructed ductal system by the radiologist. Check it out.

Surgical Strategies

If the patient is one of the majority who settles with initial conservative measures, then one can select to perform one of the following *semi-elective* procedures:

- Preoperative ERCP with common duct clearance, followed by laparoscopic cholecystectomy
- ERCP with common duct clearance alone – leaving in gallbladder *in situ*. This is indicated in the very high-risk patient; on follow-up most so treated patients never require a cholecystectomy.
- Laparoscopic cholecystectomy with laparoscopic common bile duct exploration
- Open cholecystectomy with common bile duct exploration

In most hospitals preoperative ERCP is selected because it is ubiquitously available. Further, it delineates the biliary anatomy for the surgeon if periampullary carcinoma is suspected. It also provides a preoperative reassurance that the ampulla can be cannulated in the event that it is needed postoperatively for retained stones.

Primary "Emergency" Surgical Treatment

We have encountered another subset of patients who present with rapid clinical deterioration and may even develop diffuse signs suggesting gallbladder perforation. It is this group who probably benefit from an expeditious surgery following resuscitation. The case is made more compelling if they have had a prior gastrectomy that prevents rapid cannulation for ERCP. Staged surgery, comprising initial placement of a T tube and subsequent elective cholecystectomy once the patient has settled, is a safe option to remember in this situation.

136   **Conclusions**

A concordant multidisciplinary team that understands when appropriate interventions are needed best manages acute cholangitis. Since the introduction of endoscopic management of bile duct stones, surgery is seldom required as an emergency. Removal of the gallbladder and clearance of the bile duct of all stones are the 2 goals of treatment. In the absence of stones – suspect periampullary carcinoma. When the patient is toxic and ERCP fails, or is not immediately available, do not procrastinate waiting for "re-ERCP tomorrow": operate and drain the obstructed biliary system!

17 Small Bowel Obstruction

*The only thing predictable about small bowel obstruction
is its unpredictability*

By far, the most common causes of small bowel obstruction (SBO) are postoperative adhesions and hernias. Other rarer etiologies are mechanical (bolus, malignant or inflammatory). Irreducible hernias and the differential diagnosis of early postoperative SBO versus ileus are discussed separately in chapters 18 and 34, respectively. Mention will be made below of SBO in the "virgin" abdomen. The bulk of this chapter is devoted to adhesive SBO.

The Dilemma

A significant number of SBO patients respond to conservative (non-operative) treatment. But persevering with conservative management in SBO may delay the recognition of compromised (strangulated) bowel, leading to excessive morbidity and mortality. Clearly, your challenge revolves around the following issues:

- Which patients need an urgent laparotomy for impending or established bowel strangulation? And when is initial, conservative treatment appropriate and safe?
- Once instituted, how long should conservative treatment be continued before an operation is deemed necessary? In other words, how to save the patient an operation without risking intestinal compromise?

You will be provided with guidelines to answer these questions. But first we need to re-emphasize some definitions.

138   **Definitions**

- *Simple obstruction*: the bowel is blocked from within, compressed or kinked, but its vascular supply is not threatened.
- *Strangulation- obstruction*: the vascular supply to the segment of obstructed bowel is compromised.
- *Closed loop obstruction*: there is a double obstruction in a segment of bowel at a proximal and distal point. Commonly, the involved bowel is strangulated.

Understanding the terms "*partial*" versus "*complete*" obstruction is crucial to the planning of treatment. These terms are based on plain abdomen radiographic findings:

- *Partial obstruction*: there is air present in the colon, in addition to the small bowel distention with air and fluid levels.
- *Complete obstruction*: no air seen in the colon.

Most episodes of partial SBO resolve without an operation, while the majority of patients presenting with a complete obstruction do require one.

Clinical Features

The three important clinical manifestations of SBO are colicky abdominal pain, vomiting and distension. Constipation is only a symptom of late SBO. The pattern of these features depends on the site, the cause and the duration of the obstruction. For example, in high obstruction, vomiting is prominent while pain and distension mild; as the level of obstruction descends, the crampy pain becomes more marked. In very distal SBO, distension is the outstanding symptoms with vomiting appearing only later. Feculent vomiting is usually the hallmark of long-standing, distal, complete SBO and is characteristic of massive bacterial overgrowth proximal to the obstruction (*Remember* – the main bulk of feces is made of bacteria).

The essential radiographic features on the supine and erect abdominal X rays are well-known (chapter 3): gaseous distension of the bowel proximal to the obstruction, presence of air-fluid levels and, in complete SBO, absence of gas distal to the obstruction. The presence of parallel striations (caused by the valvulae conniventes) running transversely, right across the lumen are characteristic of distended small bowel.

Is There a Strangulation?

The answer to this question is crucial: if positive, not only is an operation compulsory, it also needs to be performed with a certain degree of urgency. The most important feature of strangulation is *continuous pain*. These patients tend to become sicker more rapidly. Signs of peritoneal irritation (guarding, rebound tenderness) may be present but remember that:

- Dead bowel can be present with a relatively "innocent" abdomen.
- Signs of peritoneal irritation are rarely useful in differentiating simple obstruction from strangulation because they may also be found in simple SBO when the distension is severe.

Do not wait for fever, leukocytosis or acidosis to diagnose ischemic bowel because these systemic signs are an indication that the intestine is already dead!

Having diagnosed strangulation, you will be congratulated for having expeditiously resuscitated and wheeled your patient to the operating room. Save yourself the embarrassment of explaining, the next day, the presence of the long midline incision to deal with a knuckle of ischemic gut trapped in the groin! Never forget that the most common cause of strangulated bowel is an external hernia. The suspicion of strangulation must make you examine, or rather re-examine more carefully, the five external hernial orifices: two inguinal, two femoral and one umbilical (chapter 18).

You have to understand that: nothing, nothing can accurately distinguish between "simple" and "strangulating" SBO. So how to play it safe?

Management

Fluid and Electrolytes

There is hardly a need to remind you that SBO results in significant losses (or sequestration) of extracellular fluid and electrolytes, which have to be replaced intravenously. The aggressiveness of fluid management and hemodynamic monitoring depend on the condition of the individual patient. The fluid of choice is Ringer's lactate. The charting of urine output in a catheterized patient is the minimal monitoring necessary. Even patients scheduled for urgent laparotomy for strangulation require adequate pre-operative resuscitation (chapter 5). Patients with SBO sometimes have intra-abdominal hypertension, which may falsely raise their cardiac filling pressures (CVP, wedge). These patients require all the more aggressive fluid administration to maintain adequate cardiac output (chapter 28).

Nasogastric Aspiration

A large NG tube (at least 18F in diameter) is needed. The NG tube has both therapeutic and diagnostic functions. It controls vomiting. But its main aim is to decompress the dilated stomach and consequently the gut proximal to the obstruction, which overflows back into the stomach. In a simple obstruction, decompression of the obstructed bowel results rapidly in pain relief and alleviates the distension. In strangulation or close-loop obstruction, the pain persists despite naso-gastric aspiration.

Insertion of a NG tube is extremely unpleasant. Many patients remember it as the most horrendous experience of their hospital stay (and would certainly resist fiercely any attempt at re-insertion). The procedure can be made much "kinder": soften the rigid tube by immersion for a minute or two in hot water; spray the nostril and throat of the patient with a local anesthetic; and lubricate the tube. There is no advantage in connecting the NG tube to a suction apparatus; drainage by gravity is as effective and more "physiological". Long naso-intestinal tubes are a gimmick with unproven benefits – requiring cumbersome manipulations and causing delay when operation is necessary.

When to Operate?

The first hour or two of fluid replenishment is compulsory in the management of every patient. Re-assess your resuscitated patient: what is now the pattern of pain ? Is there improvement on abdominal re-examination?

Immediate operation is required in a minority of patients: those who do not improve, those who experience continuous pain, or those with significant abdominal tenderness. Abdominal X-rays usually show a complete obstruction. The probability of strangulation is high. Book them for an emergency operation.

An initial non-operative approach is often possible because most patients improve at first on the "drip-and-suck" regimen. It would be safe to bet, at this stage, that patients with radiological partial obstruction will eventually escape surgery while those with complete obstruction will visit, in time, the operating room. But how long is it safe to continue with conservative management? This is a controversial issue. Some surgeons would abort the conservative trial at 24 hours if the patient fails to "open up", because of the nagging concern about strangulation even in a benign-looking abdomen. Others are prepared to persevere, up to 5 days, in a carefully monitored patient. In the absence of an immediate

142 indication for operation, we favor the use of an oral water-soluble contrast medium (e.g. Gastrografin) as soon as the diagnosis of SBO is made. Gastrografin, a hyperosmolar agent that promotes intestinal "hurry", plays two roles: diagnostic-prognostic and therapeutic.

The Gastrografin "Challenge"

After the initial gastric decompression, 100 ml of Gastrografin are instilled through the NG tube, which is then clamped for 2 hours. Four to 6 hours later, a simple plain abdominal X-ray is obtained. This is not a formal radiological study under fluoroscopy. Make sure that your patient does not get barium (chapter 3). Presence of contrast in the large bowel proves that the obstruction is partial. In most these instances, the Gastrografin is passed per rectum. In partial SBO, Gastrografin is often therapeutic as it expedites the resolution of the obstructing episode. On the other hand, failure of Gastrografin to reach the colon within 6 hours indicates a complete obstruction. The probability of spontaneous resolution after a failed Gastrografin "challenge" is very low; most these patients will require surgery. However, a repeat challenge may sometimes succeed. Of course the results of the Gastrografin "challenge" test should be correlated with the whole clinical picture. Note that Gastrografin may pass across a chronic SB narrowing. Thus, for the obstructive episode to be considered as "resolved" the abdominal symptoms and signs should disappear as well.

Additional Investigations

Clinical examination and plain abdominal radiographs, complemented with a Gastrografin follow-through suffice to reach the correct decision in the majority of patients. Is additional imaging necessary? *Ultrasonography* has been reported by enthusiasts to accurately define the site of obstruction

and establish whether strangulation is present. It requires access to an   143
expert which most institutions lack. Oral and IV contrast-enhanced *CT*
has been shown an accurate modality to establish the level of obstruction
and to diagnose a strangulated bowel segment. This however does not
mean that CT is usually necessary. CT should be resorted to selectively
in the following scenarios:

- History of abdominal malignancy; a CT finding of diffuse carcinomatosis with or without ascites could imply that symptomatic
  management is the correct option.
- Clinical picture not consistent with the usual partial adhesive SBO.
  Paralytic ileus may be easily confused with a partial SBO (chapter
  35): there is air in the large bowel, the Gastrografin goes through
  but the patient remains symptomatic; fever and/or leukocytosis
  may be present. CT may document the underlying cause of
  peritonitis responsible for the paralytic ileus (e.g. appendicular or
  diverticular mass).

Antibiotics

In animal models of SBO, systemic antibiotics delay intestinal compromise
and decrease mortality. In clinical practice, there is no need for antibiotics
in patients treated conservatively, and we operate whenever the suspicion
of intestinal compromise is entertained. A single pre-operative dose of
antibiotics is administered prophylactically; no postoperative antibiotics
are necessary even if bowel resection has been performed (chapters 6 &
32). The only indication for postoperative therapeutic administration
would be long-standing bowel gangrene with established intra-abdominal
infection.

144   **The Conduct of the Operation**

- The incision for abdominal re-entry has been discussed in chapter 8 but we need to remind you to carefully avoid iatrogenic enterotomies with their associated potential postoperative morbidity. Finding your way into the peritoneal cavity may take time, but be patient for this is the longest part of the procedure. The rest is usually simpler.

- Find a loop of collapsed small bowel and follow it proximally. It will lead you to the point of obstruction just distal to the dilated-obstructed intestine. Now deal with the cause of obstruction, be it a simple band or a bowel kink. Mobilize the involved bowel segment using sharp and blunt dissection with traction applied on the two structures to be separated.

- Resect only non-viable bowel or when the obstructed segment is impossible to be freed. Frequently, an ischemic-looking loop of bowel is dusky after being released. Do not rush to resect; cover the bowel with a warm – wet laparotomy pad and wait patiently; it will usually pink up within ten minutes. If not, it requires resection.

- Concentrate on the loop, which is responsible for the obstruction; there is no need to free the whole intestine by dividing all the remaining innocent adhesions. This maneuver may be cosmetically appealing, but adhesions lysed today will re-form tomorrow. Occasionally, multiple points of obstruction appear to be present with no clear area of demarcation between dilated and collapsed bowel. This is more common in patients after multiple operations for SBO or those with early postoperative SBO. In this situation the whole length of the gut has to be unraveled.

How to manage an iatrogenic intestinal injury during adhesiolysis?
Transmural enterotomies should be repaired. We recommend a running, one-layered, absorbable, monofilament technique (chapter 11). Superficial

serosal tears should be left alone. Areas where the mucosa pouts through   145
the defect should be repaired with a running monofilament seromuscular
suture.

Decompress Or Not ?

Attempting decompression of the proximal distended bowel represents a
double edge sword. On the one hand, excessive bowel distension impedes
abdominal closure and contributes to postoperative intra-abdominal
hypertension with its well-known deleterious physiological consequences
(chapter 28). On the other hand, bowel decompression may contribute to
postoperative ileus and even cause peritoneal contamination. Most
would decompress the distended bowel by gently milking its contents
towards the stomach, from where it is sucked by the anesthetist. Milk the
bowel very gently with your index and middle fingers, as obstructed
bowel is thin-walled and very easily injured. Do not pull too hard on the
mesentery. Feel, from time to time, the stomach; if full, gently squeeze
and shake it to restore patency of the NG tube. For distal SBO, you may
also milk the small bowel contents towards the collapsed colon. Be that
as it may, "open" decompression through an enterotomy is unwise, given
the risk of gross contamination. Needle decompression is not effective,
as enteric juices are abnormally viscous. Obviously, open decompression
should be performed if bowel is being resected: insert a "pool" sucker or
a large sump drain connected to the suction through the proximal line of
bowel transection and "accordion" the bowel onto your suction device.
    Before closing, "run" the bowel again for missed enterotomies.
Check for hemostasis, as extensive adhesiolysis leaves large oozing raw
areas; and intra-peritoneal blood promotes ileus, infection and more
adhesion formation. Close the abdomen safely (chapter 29). SBO is
a risk for wound dehiscence and a "classic" for the M & M conference –
chapter 42.

146   **Special Circumstances**

The "Virgin" Abdomen

The patient presents with clinical and radiological features of SBO but with no abdominal wall scar of previous surgery. What to do? Evidence of a complete obstruction is of course an indication for a laparotomy but what with partial SBO? As with the adhesive partial obstruction, we recommend a Gastrografin "challenge". In an obstruction caused by an intraluminal bolus, be it parasites or dry fruits, Gastrografin may dis-impact the bowel. In these cases, we would recommend elective abdominal imaging to exclude an underlying cause. Non-resolving partial obstruction despite the Gastrografin "challenge", may be evidence of a mechanical cause, such as a congenital band, an internal hernia, malignancy or inflammation. Laparotomy usually uncovers a treatable cause of ob-struction. Resist the temptation to order a CT scan "just to find out what we're dealing with". It only delays the operation without changing its indication. SBO due to a previously undiagnosed but suspected Crohn's Disease is an exception; here a CT may be very suggestive – indicating continued conservative therapy (chapter 20).

The Known Cancer Patient

A patient is admitted with SBO a year or two following an operation for gastric or colonic cancer. You should first attempt to obtain information about the findings at the previous laparotomy. The more advanced the can-cer then, the higher the probability that the current obstruction is malig-nant. Clinically, cachexia, ascites or an abdominal mass suggests diffuse carcinomatosis. These cases present a medical and ethical dilemma: on the one hand, one wishes to relieve the obstruction and offer the patient a further spell of quality life. On the other hand, one tries to spare a terminal patient an unnecessary operation. Each case should be assessed on merit.

In the absence of stigmata of advanced disease, surgery for complete obstruction is justifiable. In many instances adhesions may be found; in
others, a bowel segment obstructed by local spread or metastases can be
bypassed. When diffuse carcinomatosis is suspected clinically, or on CT
scan, a reasonable option would be to insert a palliative, venting gastrostomy, allowing the patient to die peacefully at home or in a Hospice
environment.

Radiation Enteritis

Radiation treatment of abdominal or pelvic malignancies is not an
uncommon cause of SBO; this usually develops months or even years
after irradiation. A relentless course of multiple episodes of partial SBO,
initially responding to conservative treatment but eventually culminating
in a complete obstruction, is characteristic. There is also the uncertainty
about the obstruction being malignant or adhesive in nature. One always
hopes it is adhesive, because SBO due to radiation injury is "bad news"
indeed. When forced to operate for complete obstruction, one finds
irradiated loops of bowel glued or welded together and onto adjacent
structures. The paper-thin bowel tears easily. Accidental enterotomies
are frequent, difficult to repair, and commonly result in postoperative
fistulas. Short involved segments of bowel are best resected, but when
longer segments are encountered, usually stucked in the pelvis, it is safest
to bail out with an entero-enteric or entero-colic bypass. Postoperative
short- bowel syndrome is common whatever the procedure. Long-term
prognosis is poor: irradiation enteritis is almost as bad as the malignancy
the irradiation had attempted to control.

Recurrent Multiple Episodes of SBO

The patient is typically re-admitted every second month for SBO and
had undergone, in the past, multiple operations for this condition. How

148 should he be managed? We would treat him as any other patient presenting with adhesive SBO. Fortunately, most such episodes are "partial", responsive to conservative treatment. When complete obstruction develops, operative management is obviously necessary. Attempts at preventing subsequent episodes with bowel or mesentery plication or long tube stenting are recommended by some. The evidence in favor of such maneuvers is anecdotal at best. We do not practice them. Occasionally a patient develops obstruction early in the aftermath of an operation for SBO: this is a case par excellence for prolonged non-operative management, with the patient maintained on TPN until adhesions mature and the obstruction resolves as also discussed in chapter 34).

Gallstone Ileus

Gallstone ileus develops typically in elderly patients with longstanding cholelithiasis. It is caused by a large gallstone eroding into an adjacent segment of bowel – usually the duodenum – which then migrates distally, until "stranded" at the narrow ileum. Presentation is usually vague as initially the stone may dis-impact spontaneously – causing intermittent episodes of partial obstruction. You will never miss the diagnosis once you habitually and obsessively search for *air in the bile ducts* on any plain abdominal X ray you order. The air enters the bile duct via the entero-cholecystic fistula created by the eroding gallstone. Treatment is operative and should be tailored to the condition of the patient. In frail and sick patients deal only with the SBO: place an enterotomy proximal to the stone and remove it; search for additional stones in the bowel above – you do not want to have to re-operate! In patients who are reasonably fit and well you should also deal with the cause of the problem – the gallbladder. Perform a cholecystectomy and close the duodenal defect.

Prognosis

Overall, more than half the patients presenting with an adhesive SBO can be managed without an operation. About half the patients will suffer subsequent episodes of SBO, irrespective of the treatment – surgical or conservative. *The aim is therefore to operate only when necessary but not to delay a necessary operation.*

18 "Acute" Abdominal Wall Hernias

There is no doubt that the first appearance of the mammal,
with his unexplained need to push his testicles
out of their proper home into the air,
made a mess of the three layered abdomen that had
done the reptiles well for 200 million years"
(Sir Heneage Ogilvie)

In the Western world many more hernias are now repaired electively than was formerly the case. In spite of this, the acute presentation of groin hernias to emergency surgeons remains a common occurrence and it is important to know how to deal with them.

A word about terminology: groin hernias, inguinal or femoral, may be described as reducible, irreducible, incarcerated, strangulated, obstructed. This terminology can be confusing and the words, which have come to mean different things to different people, are much less important than the concepts, which underlie the recognition and management of acute hernia problems. The important concept to be grasped is that any hernia, which becomes painful, tense, inflamed, tender and is not readily reducible should be regarded as a surgical emergency.

Presentation

Essentially patients may present acutely in one of two ways:
- Symptoms and signs related directly to the hernia itself.
- Abdominal symptoms and signs, which at first may not seem to be related to a hernia.

The first mode of presentation usually means pain and tenderness in the irreducible and tense hernia. A hernia, which was reducible, may suddenly become irreducible. The problem is obvious.

The second method of presentation may be much more insidious. Beware of the vomiting old lady! Treated at home for several days by the primary care physician as a case of gastro-enteritis she eventually comes under the care of the surgeons due to intractable emesis. By this stage she is dehydrated and in need of much resuscitation. It is surprisingly easy in these circumstances to miss the small femoral hernia barely palpable in the groin. A knuckle of small bowel is just sufficiently trapped to cause obstruction. No abdominal symptoms or signs are present and the plain abdominal radiographs are non-diagnostic. None of these difficulties saves you from the embarrassment of the following morning's round when the hernia is discovered.

Hernias are still one of the commonest causes of small bowel obstruction (chapter 17). A careful search must be made for them in all cases of actual or suspected intestinal obstruction. This may mean meticulous, prolonged and disagreeable palpation of groins, which have not seen the light of day, let alone soap and water for a long time. In most cases however the diagnosis is obvious with a classical bowel obstruction and a hernia stuck in the scrotum. Beware of the *Richter's* hernia – typical to the femoral hernia, where only a portion of the circumference of the bowel is strangulated. Because the intestinal lumen is not completely blocked, presentation is delayed and non-specific.

Preparation

As we suggested earlier, some patients may be in need of quite a bit of resuscitation on admission to the hospital. Surgery for acute groin hernia problems should be carried out without undue delay, but nevertheless these patients must not be rushed to surgery without careful assessment and preparation (chapter 5). Analgesia is an important part of the management of these patients. Opiate analgesia and bed rest with the foot of the bed slightly elevated may successfully manage a painful obstructed hernia of short duration. Gentle attempts at reduction of such a hernia are justified once the analgesics have taken effect. A successful reduction of the hernia means that emergency surgery at unsociable hours may be traded for a semi-elective procedure on the next available routine list – a benefit for both patient and surgeon. Note that manual reduction of the incarcerated hernia should be attempted only in the absence of signs of intestinal strangulation; it should be gently performed, to avoid *"reduction en masse"* – when the herniated bowel with the constricting ring are reduced together, with persisting symptoms of strangulation.

The Operation

Inguinal Hernia

An inguinal incision is a satisfactory approach. Even if a bowel resection is required it is possible to deliver sufficient length of intestine through the inguinal canal to carry this out.

The main difference in dissection in an emergency hernia operation compared to an elective procedure is in the moment at which the hernial sac is opened. In the emergency situation the hernia will often reduce spontaneously as soon as the constricting ring is divided. The site of constriction may be the superficial inguinal ring, in which case the hernia reduces when external oblique is opened. It is recommended therefore that the sac is opened and the contents grasped for later inspection before the constricting tissues are released. If the hernia reduces before the sac contents are inspected it is important that they are subsequently identified and retrieved so that a loop of non-viable gut is not left in the abdomen. Retrieval of reduced sac contents can be an awkward business via the internal ring and occasionally a formal laparotomy may be required to inspect matters properly. It is for these reasons that great care should be

154   taken to retain the sac contents for inspection as soon as possible during the procedure.

If the hernial sac contains omentum only, then any tissue which is necrotic or of doubtful viability should be excised, ensuring meticulous hemostasis in the process. If on the other hand bowel is involved, then any areas of questionable viability should be wrapped in a warm moist gauze pack and left for a few minutes to recover. Irreversibly ischemic gut should be resected. If there is a small patch of necrosis which does not involve the whole circumference of the bowel then this can sometimes be dealt with by invagination rather than by resorting to resection. In this situation the injured bowel wall is invaginated by a seromuscular suture, taking bites on the viable bowel on either side of the defective area of gut.

Occasionally, particularly if a bowel resection has been necessary, edema of the herniated gut makes its replacement into the abdomen difficult. Manoeuvres such as putting the patient into a marked Trendelenburg position and gently compressing the eviscerated gut, covered by a large moist gauze swab, will invariably allow the bowel to be replaced in the abdomen. It is possible to minimise the chances of this difficulty arising if care is taken during any bowel resection not to have any more gut outside the abdomen than is absolutely necessary. Very rarely the herniated viscera won't return into the abdomen without pulling on it from *within*. In such instance La Rocque's manoeuvre may be useful: extend the skin incision up and laterally; then split the external oblique aponeurosis and follow this with a muscle splitting incision of internal oblique and transverse muscles above the internal ring. Through this incision you enter the peritoneal cavity and reduce the hernial contents simply by pulling on it from within.

The question of the type of hernia repair to be employed is a matter for the individual surgeon, with one proviso. In these days of tension free hernia repair it seems imprudent to place large amounts of mesh in the groin if necrotic gut has had to be resected. In this situation some other type of repair seems advisable to obviate the misery of infected mesh.

Femoral Hernia

Essentially you can approach the acute femoral hernia from below the inguinal canal, from above, or through it.

- With the *low approach*, you place the incision below the inguinal ligament – directly over the bulge. You find the hernial sac and open it – making sure to grasp its contents for proper inspection. Strangulated omentum may be excised, viable bowel is reduced back into the peritoneal cavity through the femoral ring. When the ring is tight, and usually it is – you can stretch it with your small finger, inserted medially to the femoral vein. You can resect non-viable small bowel through this approach and even anastomose its ends, but pushing the sutured or stapled anastomosis back into the abdomen is like trying to squeeze a tomato into a cocktail glass. Therefore, when bowel has to be resected it is advisable to do it through a small right lower quadrant muscle splitting laparotomy (as for appendectomy).

- Some authorities favour an approach *via the inguinal canal* but we can see little merit in this approach which must disrupt the anatomy of the canal and presumably risk subsequent inguinal hernias.

- Yet another approach is the McEvedy's. This involves an approach to the extraperitoneal space along the lateral border of the lower part of rectus abdominis. The skin incision may be vertical, in line with the border of rectus, or oblique/horizontal. A vertical skin incision has the merit of allowing extension to a point below the inguinal ligament and this may be helpful in reducing stubborn hernias, allowing traction from above and compression from below. Once the space behind rectus muscle has been accessed the hernia can usually be freed from behind the inguinal ligament. The peritoneum can be opened as widely as necessary to permit inspection of the contents of the hernial sac and to carry out intestinal resection if necessary.

156   All above approaches are reasonable provided the contents of the hernial
sac are examined and dealt with appropriately. As with inguinal hernias
the implantation of large amounts of mesh should be avoided in patients
who have contamination of the operative field with intestinal contents.
With this caveat the choice of repair is not different from what you
would do in the elective situation.

Incisional Hernias

Incisional hernias are common but most are asymptomatic except the
unsightly bulge and discomfort they often produce. It is the small
incisional henias with the tight neck, which become acutely symptomatic –
incarcerating omentum or intestine.

The presentation is well known to you: an old "silent" hernia or abdominal scar, which has become now painful. When bowel is incarcerated
there may be associated symptoms of SBO (chapter 17). The hernia itself
is tense, tender and non-reducible. It is important to distinguish between
intestinal obstruction *caused* by the incisional hernia or simply *associated*
with it. The latter situation, which is not uncommon, implies that the
patient suffers SBO caused by adhesions for example, and the obstructed
and distended loops of bowel invade the long-standing incisional hernia.
On examination, the bowel-filled tender hernia may mimic incarceration.
It is for this reason that the contents of any hernia associated with
obstruction must be carefully examined at operation to ensure that the
hernia truly is the cause of the obstruction.

Any acute incisional hernia is a surgical emergency. This is also
true with other types of abdominal wall hernias – such as the umbilical
or epigastric ones. At operation the hernial sac has to be entered to
evaluate the incarcerated contents which are to be reduced or resected
depending on the findings. *The surgical findings should explain the clinical
presentation.* For example: if you do not find strangulated omentum or
bowel in the sac you have to retrieve the whole length of the intestine

in search for distal SBO. If you find pus within the sac you have to look   157
for the source. We have seen patients operated upon for a "strangulated
incisional hernia" when the underlying diagnosis was perforated appendicitis.

   After the contents of the hernia have been dealt, with identify the
fascial margins of the defect. Use your conventional "best" repair but do
not forget that placing a mesh in a contaminated field is potentially
problematic. In critically ill patient, when the repair deems complex or is
judged to significantly increase the intra-abdominal pressure – we would
simply close the skin – leaving the patient with a large incisional hernia.
*Remember – patients do not die form the hernia itself but from its intesti-
nal complications or a too tight closure* (chapters 28 & 29).

   **You can judge the worth of a surgeon by the way he does a hernia.
   (Fairbank)**

19 Acute Mesenteric Ischemia

*Severe abdominal pain out of proportion to findings on examination –
think about acute mesenteric ischemia*

The Problem

The problem is a sudden reduction in arterial perfusion of the small
bowel, which results in an immediate central abdominal pain. If left
untreated, the process involves progressively the muscular layer of the
intestines and only when, after hours, the serosa is affected peritoneal
signs appear. To simplify matters let us divide acute mesenteric ischemia
to three types which are almost equally common:

- *Thrombotic*: due to an acute arterial thrombosis which occludes
  usually the orifice of the superior mesenteric artery (SMA),
  resulting in massive ischemia of the entire small bowel plus the
  right colon – the area supplied by the SMA.
- *Embolic*: due to a shower of embolic material originating proximally – from the heart (atrial fibrillation, post MI, diseased valve) or
  an aneurysmal or atherosclerotic aorta. Emboli lodge usually at the
  proximal SMA, but below the entry of the middle colic artery;
  therefore – as a rule – the most proximal segment of proximal SB is
  spared. Emboli tend also to fragment – and re-emboli distally – producing a patchy type, small bowel ischemia.
- *Non-occlusive*: due to "low flow state", in the absence of documented
  arterial thrombosis or embolus. Note, however, that an underlying
  mesenteric atherosclerosis may be a precipitating – contributory
  factor. The low flow state is a product of low cardiac output (e.g.
  cardiogenic shock), reduced mesenteric flow (e.g. intra-abdominal
  hypertension) or mesenteric vasoconstriction (e.g. administration
  of vasopressors) – usually, however, due to a combination of these
  factors, developing in the settings of pre-existent critical illness.

160   *Mesenteric Venous Thrombosis* can also produce small bowel ischemia. The features and management of this entity differs drastically from the above mentioned three. It will be discussed separately below.

The problem is that in clinical practice, outside the textbook, mesenteric ischemia is usually recognized when it has already led to intestinal gangrene. At such a time the Pandora's Box of SIRS has been opened and even removal of the entire gangrenous intestine will not stop the progression to organ failure and death. Even if such physiologic consequences can be overcome the patient commonly becomes an "intestinal cripple" – suffering from short bowel syndrome.

Assessing the Problem

Typically, the early clinical picture is non-specific: *the patient complains of severe abdominal pain – if he is able to complain at all – and the doctor finds little on physical examination.*

There may have been preceding symptoms of a similar sort of pain developing with meals and accompanied by weight loss – suggesting pre-existing *mesenteric angina*. History or evidence of systemic atherosclerotic vascular disease is almost the rule in patients with mesenteric thrombosis while a source for emboli, such as atrial fibrillation, is usually present in patients with mesenteric embolism. Low flow state patients are commonly moribund due to underlying critical disease.

Nausea, vomiting, diarrhea and hematochezia come late if ever. You must resist the natural temptation to ascribe patients' non-specific symptoms to some other benign condition such as gastroenteritis unless the associated history and symptoms for the alternate explanation are fully present. And by the way – in the elderly – the diagnosis of "acute gastroenteritis" very rarely is the *final* diagnosis.

Physical examination in the early stages of the process is treacherously benign – peritoneal irritation appearing as a rule when it is too late and the bowel is dead.

Plain abdominal x-rays early in the course of the illness are normal. 161
Later there may be a pattern of adynamic ileus, with visible loops of
small bowel and air/fluid levels, but with gas and feces seen within the
normal colon and rectum. Likewise, *laboratory studies* usually are normal
until the intestine loses viability; only then do leukocytosis, hyperamyle-
semia, and lactic acidosis develop.

The bottom line is that initially in acute mesenteric ischemia the
physical examination and all commonly available x-rays and blood tests
are *normal*. At this stage, entertaining the diagnosis of mesenteric ischemia,
you have two options: the first is to enter in the chart: "abdominal
examination normal; mesenteric ischemia cannot be ruled out; will
re-assess later". The second option is to order a mesenteric angiogram.
Unfortunately, the first option is the still prevailing one in the community –
leading to procrastination, late diagnosis and treatment, and a very high
mortality rate.

Mesenteric Angiography

To be beneficial the angiogram should be performed ASAP. The clock is
tickling; any minute passing reduces the chances of the bowel and the
patient. Note that an "acute abdomen" with peritoneal signs is a contraindication for angiography. The radiologist should start with a biplaner
angiography (i.e. including a later view to show the origin of the SMA
and the celiac axis). *Occluded ostium of the SMA* denotes thrombosis and
calls for an immediate operation – unless there is an evidence for a good
collateral inflow – the angiography providing the road map for vascular
reconstruction. When the ostium is patent the radiologist advances the
catheter into the SMA. *Emboli* lodge distally to the takeoff of the middle
colic artery, produce a smooth filling defect on the background of
normal SMA, and can be multiple.

162   Non-operative Treatment

In the absence peritoneal signs attempts at non-operative treatment are justified – tailored to the clinical/angiographic scenario.

The selective diagnostic angiography can now become therapeutic – infusing a thrombolytic agent to lyse the thrombus or embolus with or without adding papaverine to relieve the associated mesenteric vasospasm. Cessation of abdominal symptoms together with angiographic resolution means that the emergency is over; preexisting mesenteric artery stenoses can be addressed electively – if indicated.

In the event of *non-occlusive* mesenteric ischemia the approach involves attempts at restoring altered hemodynamics. To relieve associated arteriospasm, a selective intra-arterial infusion of a vasodilator medication, such as papaverine, has been advocated. The few champions of the method reported "favorable response". When *emboli* are the cause, after successful trans-catheter therapy long-term anticoagulation is indicated. A final point: while rushing to the arteriography suit remember to adequately hydrate your patient to oppose the nephrotoxic potentials of the contrast media to be used in large quantities.

Operative Treatment

As we told you above – peritoneal signs is an indication *not* to do an arteriography but to operate; the same applies to the failure of non-operative regimen discussed above. Through midline incision assess the viability of the intestine. In general there are two main possible scenario: the one is the bowel *being frankly gangrenous* ("dead"), the second when the bowel "appears ischemic" ("dusky") and of questionable viability.

Frank Gangrene

Frank gangrene of the entire small bowel is usually combined with the same fate of the right colon and signifies SMA thrombosis. Theoretically, a sporadic patient could survive the resection of his entire small bowel and right colon. He may even tolerate a duodenocolic anastomosis while nutritionally supported at home with total parenteral nutrition (TPN). But the eventual mortality of such an "exercise', in the average elderly vasculopath, is approaching 100% and the cost is immense. Our recommendation to you when involved in a similar scenario: walk out to talk to the family, explain that anything done will only increase the suffering of their beloved one, return and close the abdomen over the dead bowel. Provide a lot of morphine and comfort.

Frank gangrene of a shorter segment of small bowel or multiple segments-usually denotes embolism. After excising all dead segments carefully examine the remaining bowel. Measure it: how long it is? Only about half of patients left with less than 1 meter (3 feet) of small bowl will live without TPN (saving the ileocecal valve improves the prognosis). Now, observe the remaining bowel: is it truly non-compromised – are the mesenteric arcades pulsating well? Feel the SMA at it's root – is it vigorously pulsating?

Dusky Bowel

When you are not happy with the remaining bowel – or when the bowel is not dead but appears ischemic and of questionable viability from the start, proceed as following: pack the bowel in warm, saline- moistened sponges and wait 15 minutes. Failure of the bowel to pink-up mandates its resection. When the length of remaining normal-looking bowel approaches is less than 1.5 meter (5 feet) it may be advisable to leave the "doubtful" bowel in situ, to be re-examined during a re-look operation

164 (see below). Saving even a short segment of SB may improve the chances of a reasonable life quality. Some authors recommend the use of hand-held Doppler to examine the perfusion of the anti-mesenteric side of the bowel; others use intra-operative fluorescein angiography. You may chose using such modalities if available to you but your clinical judgement may be just as good.

Adjunctive Vascular Procedures

The ideal setting to surgically improve the perfusion of small bowel is when the operation follows an emergency arteriography (plus failed angiographic therapy) and the bowel is viable or "doubtful". Obviously, when the bowel is dead – it cannot be revived! Arteriography serves a road map: when the SMA is occluded – thrombosed at its origin – a vein or graft bypass, antegrade or retrograde, is indicated to re-perfuse the SMA. Such scenario is however extremely rare; more commonly you'll encounter a picture of SMA embolism: palpate for the SMA just at the base of the mesocolon – if non pulsatile you'll find it, after incising the peritoneum, to the right of the large/blue-SMV. After obtaining control, open the artery transversely and pass up and down a small Fogarty embolectomy balloon catheter. You may conclude the procedure with a shot of urokinase injected distally to lyse the clots in the side brunches, which are inaccessible to your embolectomy balloon catheter.

To Anastomose or Not?

You should be very *selective* in attempting an anastomosis following the resection of devitalized intestine. The patient has to be hemodynamically stable and his nutritional status at least fair. To be hooked-up the remaining bowel has to be of non-questionable viability and the peritoneal

cavity free of "established" infection. Most crucially, the cause of ischemia
has to be "solved". Another factor strongly bearing on your decision is
the length of the remaining bowel and its predicted postoperative
function. When more than half of the SB are resected – the resection is
considered "massive". Restoring intestinal continuity in such cases
would lead to poorly tolerable and intractable diarrhea. And finally, the
chief reason not to anastomose the bowel is the possibility that further
ischemia may develop.

We recommend, therefore, that whenever the above mentioned
factors are absent, or when resection is "massive", the two ends of the
resected bowel are to be exteriorized as an end-enterostomy and mucous
fistula – if possible via one abdominal wall site (this would allow a subsequent re-anastomosis without a major laparotomy). The postoperative
appearance of the stomas will accurately reflect the status of the remaining
bowel.

Second-Look Operations?

A routine planned "second-look" re-operation allows direct re-assessment
of intestinal viability at the earliest possible stage, before additional
mediators of SIRS have been released, and in a way which aims to preserve
the greatest possible length of viable intestine. This concept, which in
theory at least is attractive, motivates many surgeons to re-explore their
patients routinely after 24 to 48 hours. The finding of completely normal
bowel at re-operation is of course reassuring but the anastomosis may
still leak five days after it has been observed to be intact. If you plan a
"second look" operation there is no need to close the abdomen at the
end of the first procedure; instead, treat the abdomen as a laparostomy
(chapter 37) until re-exploration – relieving the intra-abdominal hypertension to further improve mesenteric blood flow.

Another alternative option is to close the abdomen, leaving a few laparoscopic ports adjacent to the bowel, through which subsequently a laparoscope is inserted to assess the status of the bowel.

To sum-up – it appears that in most patients who at the end of the operation do not have stomas, a second-look procedure is indicated. Those with viable stomas and otherwise "well" can be observed.

Mesenteric Venous Thrombosis

This is a rare condition, which occludes the venous outflow of the bowel. Clinical presentation is entirely non-specific, with abdominal pain and varying gastrointestinal symptoms, which may last a few days until eventually the intestine are compromised and peritoneal signs develop. Mesenteric venous thrombosis may be idiopathic (e.g. – the doctor is an idiot – ignorant of the underlying reason) but commonly an underlying hypercoagulable state (such as polycytemia vera) or sluggish portal flow due to hepatic cirrhosis, are present.

Typically, many of these patients are admitted to "medicine" with a surgeon consulted only late – to operate for non-viable bowel. However, an early trip to a contrast-enhanced CT scan may achieve an earlier diagnosis, helping to avoid an operation all together and improve survival. Characteristic findings on CT represent a *triad* of:

- A hypodensity in the trunk of the SMV
- Associated intra-peritoneal fluid
- Thickened segment of SB

With the above findings, and in the absence of peritoneal signs, full systemic anticoagulation with heparin may result in a spontaneous resolution of the process. The role of systemic thrombolysis is not clear. Failure to improve or peritoneal signs mandate an operation.

At surgery, you'll find some free sero-sanguineous peritoneal fluid;   167
the small bowel will be thick, edematous, dark-blue but not frankly
"dead", with the involved intestinal segment poorly demarcated. Arterial
pulsations will be present and thrombosed veins seen. You'll need to
resect the affected bowel; whether to anastomose or not and considerations about the need for a "second look" – apply the same judgement as
discussed above for arterial ischemia. Postoperative anticoagulation is
mandatory to prevent progression of the thrombosing process. Adding a
venous thrombectomy is advocated by some, so is intra-operative thrombolysis; the real benefits of these controversial approaches are unknown.

Conclusion

It appears that in most places the mortality rate of acute mesenteric
ischemia is still prohibitive. Why? Because surgeons *fail* to do the
following:
- Suspect ischemia before intestinal gangrene develop.
- Proceed with diagnostic/therapeutic angiography.
- Improve intestinal perfusion during laparotomy.
- Exteriorize the bowel or execute a 'second look' operations.

If you wish to see survivors of this horrendous condition – be aggressive.

> **It is almost impossible to further increase the current M & M associated
> with acute mesenteric ischemia**

20 Inflammatory Bowel Disease

When an internist wants you to urgently operate
on his IBD patient assume
that the operation was indicated at least a week ago...

Ulcerative colitis (UC) is a disease of the colonic mucosa only. *Crohn's Disease* (CD) involves all layers of the bowel and can appear anywhere along the intestinal tract. Because of this difference UC is curable with proctocolectomy while CD is not amenable to surgical cure. For CD surgical excision of the affected bowel segment serves only to reduce symptoms, as nearly all patients will recur. The need for an emergency surgery in IBD patients has drastically diminished in recent years because patients are diagnosed earlier and better controlled by gastro-enterologists. In places where specialized care of IBD is lagging behind, emergency surgery is more common.

About a third of UC patients will eventually require an operation while nearly all with CD will have one or more operations during their lifetime. Most general surgeons will not attend more than a few cases per year and patients may be referred too late – unless gastroenterologists and surgeons cooperate and share a common philosophy of what medical and surgical treatments can and should provide. Gastroenterologists should know and appreciate that skilled surgery has a high rate of success when medical treatment fails. But surgeons must appreciate that an operation may cripple the patients and turn some into intestinal invalids.

Acute Attack of UC

There was a time when mortality was high for acute attacks of UC – both with medical and surgical treatment. It was British gastroenterologists

170   and surgeons who led the way to almost abolish mortality by establishing criteria to measure the severity of the attack and timing for operation. *The simple wisdom is that failure of medical treatment should be recognized early – being an indication for surgical treatment.* Another development has almost abolished emergency colectomy for UC as we now are able to schedule the colectomy semi-electively for nearly every patient. The skilled gastroenterologist is able to decide early when medical treatment is failing and the colectomy can then be discussed with the patient without haste. This is the standard of care the surgeon should opt for. Thus, the need for an emergency colectomy for UC in your practice implies a failure on the part of the treating team.

Assessment of the Acute UC Patient

When asked to review a case of acute UC for colectomy you should consider the following:

- *How extensive is the colitis and how badly is the mucosa affected?* The acute attack has usually been progressing since several weeks. The patient was treated ambulatory with oral steroids, then admitted to hospital and given parenteral steroids because of deterioration. Some gastroenterologists are unwilling to do a full colonoscopy for an acute attack – fearing the risk of perforation. However, a sigmoidoscopy suffices to demonstrate ulcerations. From plain abdominal films it is often possible to tell how extensive the colitis is, by demonstrating no bowel contents in the affected colon. A little air injected through a rectal catheter will function as a contrast medium – giving a good demonstration of the extent of the colitis and often disclosing the presence of ulcerations. The so-called *toxic megacolon* – an extreme dilatation and impending perforation of the colon with systemic toxicity – is a problem of the past. It should never be allowed to happen in a patient under proper

Table 20.1. Grading of ulcerative colitis

	Mild/moderate colitis	Severe colitis
Temperature	<38 C	>38 C
Pulse	<90/min	>90/min
Diarrhea	Five per day or less	Six per day or more
Blood in stool	None or little	Large amounts
Anemia	None or mild	Severe (75% or less)
Albumin	>3 g/l	<3 g/l
Abdominal pain	None or some	Severe

care, where an operation will have been scheduled long before such destruction of the colon has happened.

- *How the colonic pathology has affected the patient's physiology?* Colitis restricted to the left colon usually produces minor signs of systemic inflammation and wasting. Most such patients are not candidates for surgery unless it is obvious that the colitis cannot be controlled after extensive medical treatment has failed. We have seen however acute attacks limited to the left colon causing perforation of the sigmoid colon. In general, the extent and severity of colitis correlate with the physiological derangement of the patient. There will be fever, leukocytosis, and increased concentrations of C-reactive protein. The hemoglobin and albumin may drop significantly, often just over a few days. The patient has deteriorated while on high parenteral dose of steroids and now his physiology is breaking down. It is time to decide on the operation. Table 20.1 will allow you to better distinguish between mild/moderate colitis and a severe one – which should be taken seriously. The APACHE II score is also useful to estimate the severity of illness in this situation (chapter 5).

172 • *Are there complications of colitis?* We pay little attention to the
        number of bowel movements because the actual counts are so
        dependent on tenesmus and urgency. There are patients who have
        twenty or more bowel movements per day because of the urgency
        but the more common figure is around ten. Blood in the stools is
        common but try to get some objective information about how
        often and how much and compare with the hemoglobin concentra-
        tion. Is the patient able to compensate for the blood loss? If not – it
        strengthens the indication to operate. The bleeding that requires
        several blood transfusions is an indication for urgent colectomy;
        fortunately this has become very rare today. Considering that there
        may be extensive ulcerations of the mucosa it is remarkable that
        systemic sepsis with positive blood cultures is relatively rare.
        Associated pneumonia is occasionally present. With secondary
        infections there is no haste as it is better to treat the infection with
        antibiotics and do the colectomy a few days later. We have seen
        several cases manifesting venous thrombembolic phenomena. One
        should probably view such complications as indications that the
        host defenses and homeostasis are breaking down and that colec-
        tomy is necessary. Thrombosis and especially thrombembolism is
        a troublesome complication as its treatment with heparin may
        increase the bleeding from the bowel and the colectomy in itself is
        a distinct risk factor for further thrombembolism.

     • *The general status of the patient?* One must evaluate how the colitis
        and its treatment have affected the patient over an extended period
        of time. It should be unusual to find obvious stigmata of cortisone
        treatment apart from some edema and acne. If there is a moon
        face, muscle atrophy, hip adiposity and cutaneous striae, the patient
        has either been treated too long or is too sensitive to cortisone.
        Any such patient, in our mind, should have a colectomy to get him
        off steroids. How alert is the patient? Is he out of bed, reading or
        watching TV? At the first consultation the patient may deny the

operation as an alternative but as soon as the malaise associated
with the disease activity appears, the patient is usually happy to
consent to the operation. Both the short term and the long-term
consequences of the colitis should be considered: *the worse the
previous course has been – the stronger the indication for a colectomy
during the current attack.*

- *The nutritional status of the patient.* Withholding food and drink
  does not improve the acute attack but eating increases the diarrhea
  and most patients are unable to eat properly in the later stages of
  an acute attack. In general, in IBD patients, enteral nutrition is
  preferred over the parenteral route but total parenteral nutrition
  may be indicated in the setting of severe attack prior to the
  operation.

The Operation For Acute Colitis

Schedule the operation for the next day if the patient is in reasonably
good condition but do not delay it further. No pre-operative bowel
preparation is necessary. Antithrombotic prophylaxis with low molecular
weight heparin should be given as for elective operations. Single dose
antibiotic prophylaxis is adequate. Do not forget to "cover" the peri-
operative phase with hydrocortisone.

The operation for acute colitis is *total abdominal colectomy*: in
younger or leaner patients the colectomy is easy and should take about
2 hours; in middle aged male it can be substantially more difficult. There
are often only minor signs of inflammation on the exterior of the colon;
there may be some thickening of the wall and tortuous inflammatory
capillaries on its surface. The segmental blood vessels may be enlarged
due to the rich blood flow. You can begin the dissection on the right or
left side as is convenient. Incise the peritoneal reflections laterally and
identify the plane between the mesocolon and the retroperitoneal fascia.

174   Divide the gastrocolic ligament so the omentum is removed with the colon but the gastroepiploic artery is preserved for the stomach. Once the colon has been freed laterally it is time to divide the segmental arteries. Divide the ileum about 5 cm from the ileocolic and the rectosigmoid junction just above the promontory with the linear stapler. The closed terminal ileum is brought out through an ostomy – hole through the rectus abdominis muscle on the right side. The site should have been marked before the operation. Close the abdomen and then fashion the ostomy. Cut the bowel 5 cm above the skin, evert and suture to the skin – which results in a 2.5 cm long ileostomy.

A proctocolectomy for an acute attack of ulcerative colitis belongs to history. The remaining in situ inflamed rectum is too small to keep the patient sick. After the operation the diverted rectum becomes silent.

Your patient may be young and relatively well and the operation may appear a "piece of cake" to you. But resist the temptation to do anything more than a total abdominal colectomy – such as adding an ileorectal anastomosis of even a restorative pouch ileoproctostomy. Those patients are catabolic and on steroids – the punishment for anastomotic complications are extremely high!

Emergency Surgery for Crohn's

The need for an emergency operation in Crohn's Disease (CD) should be rare indeed. There are a few patients with acute colitis, which is clinically indistinguishable from acute ulcerative colitis (US). They are handled as acute colitis. Most of the time, however, the course and anatomical appearance of the colitis suggest that it is CD rather than UC. When small bowel is involved a diagnosis of CD is obvious. Surgery for CD demands a lot more consideration because the patient will not be cured and choosing the operation and its timing makes a difference to the future course. There is a growing understanding that repeated surgery contributes,

and perhaps is the major factor behind the phenomenon of "CD cripples"
and, even, the premature death of patients with this disease. It seems that
patients with recurrent or chronic symptomatic CD, like patients with
chronic arthritis, slowly waste over the years, to which steroids and
repeated "amputations" of bowel contribute. For those of us that believe
that any operation marks the patient permanently, biologically and socially,
it is a cause of concern that some patients with CD will have many
operations during their life. It must be stressed, however, that for the vast
majority of the cohort, timely surgery is part of the optimal treatment.
There are a few other instances, excluding acute colitis, when emergency
surgery is considered in CD patients: suspected appendicitis, small bowel
obstruction and intra-abdominal abscess.

Acute Appendicitis

If you operate for suspected acute appendicitis (chapter 22) and encounter
changes that are compatible with CD of the terminal ileum and cecum –
(e.g. serosal inflammation, thickened mesentery) what then? If the
cecum is involved but the appendix appears normal the best option is
probably to leave it alone as appendectomy may result in an entero-
cuntaneous fistula. The patient is then treated with steroids. An ileocecal
resection at that situation may provide you with the histological diagnosis
but is essentially unnecessary or could have been postponed for several
years. Almost every patient with an ileocolic resection will develop
recurrent Chron's inflammation of the anastomosis, usually within a
year, yet another reason not to be blasé about the resection. Let's not
forget that CD patients may develop acute appendicitis – which is treated
with an appendectomy.

176   Small Bowel Obstruction (SBO)

SBO is common in patients with CD. Usually it is due to a narrow segment of diseased terminal ileum but it may be caused by a more proximal stricture. When the diagnosis of CD is known you should treat the obstructive episode conservatively: SBO in CD is usually "partial" and resolves spontaneously – at least until the next exacerbation. In the absence of a previous history of CD a careful history may reveal the typical previous abdominal symptoms and systemic signs of inflammation that are compatible with a diagnosis of CD. Conservative management of SBO is discussed in chapter 17

If you operate for SBO and find an inflamed and thickened terminal ileum – picture compatible with CD; what then? It is much better and simpler to operate on CD in the elective situation – when the bowel is empty and its inside can be inspected for strictures with intraoperative endoscopy. But now the bowel is obstructed and distended. "Run" the bowel to identify any skip lesion that is more proximal and make sure there is a "passage" through them – e.g. – it is non-obstructing. Record any proximal skip lesion in your notes but leave them untouched. Your task is to deal with the acute SBO. Obstruction in CD is very rarely "complete" or "strangulating" (chapter 17); therefore, your best option is to close up the abdomen and start the patient on steroids – thus, sparing his bowel.

Rarely you'll be called to operate upon an acutely obstructed patient who failed conservative treatment: here the operative options are: resection of the ileocecal region, stricturoplasty or a temporary proximal loop-ileostomy. When the later option is adopted the inflammation is medically treated until the acute phase resolves and an elective operation can deal permanently with the affected bowel.

Intra-Abdominal Abscess

This represents a more serious pathology. There is rarely a need for emergency surgery and it is better to "convert" the acute situation to a semi-elective case. Most abdominal abscesses in CD patients can be drained percutaneously (chapter 35). The patient is then treated with antibiotics, steroids and nutritional support to allow the resolution of the acute phase before undergoing elective resection of the involved bowel – the source of the infection. Complex abscesses, which fail percutaneous drainage, should be operated upon: the involved segment of bowel has to be resected. Whether to restore bowel continuity with an anastomosis, or exteriorize the bowel end as a double-barrel stoma, depends on the condition of the patient, his abdomen and the bowel (chapter 11).

Clostridium difficile Colitis

This is not considered an IBD but is an acute colitis. With the prevalent over-use and mis-use of antimicrobial agents by physicians and surgeons *Clostridium difficile* colitis (CDC) is a common problem in hospitalized patients. CDC classically presents with diarrhea and abdominal pain following a history of antibiotic intake, with independent risk factors including age over 65, cephalosporin use, use of multiple antibiotics, prolonged hospital stay, and use of antibiotics for more than 7 days. In fact, the more antibiotics you give – the higher is the chance of the patient to develop CDC, but it can develop even after one dose. The tragedy is that patients may be dying from CDC after having received antibiotics for dubious indications.

The clinical spectrum of CDC is broad – ranging from mild diarrhea on one side, to colonic perforation of the other. The "gold standard" for diagnosis is the stool cytotoxin assay for toxin B; however the test-results may take 1–3 days. Therefore, many institutions use the latex agglutination test, which has a faster return time but is less sensitive. Bedside fibro-optic sigmoidoscopy, demonstrating the typical pseudo-membrane and ulceration is an excellent test. The preferred medical therapy for CDC includes oral metronidazole or oral vancomycin and, if the patient is unable to take oral medications, IV metronidazole. These therapies are highly effective in most patients with only a minority requiring eventually surgical therapy. Established indications for laparotomy in CDC patients include systemic deterioration and peritonitis despite optimal medical therapy.

Another subgroup of CDC patients present from the beginning with an "acute abdomen", exposing them to a highly morbid and unnecessary exploratory laparotomy which discloses viable and not perforated CDC. Therefore, remember that in any patient who presents with an "acute abdomen", with a history of recent or current antibiotic intake, and without findings which mandate an immediate exploration (e.g. free air) – CDC should be urgently excluded. Timely diagnosis of CDC through the use of sigmoidoscopy and/or CT scan – showing diffuse colonic wall thickening and colonic dilation – will allow adequate medical treatment and could spare the critically ill patient an unnecessary and risky operation.

At operation for fulminant CDC, which failed conservative treatment, the bowel appears gray and paper thin; "sealed" mini-perforations may be present. There is no doubt that subtotal colectomy is the procedure of choice when the colon is non-viable or perforated. It is also a reasonable option, albeit unproven, when operating on a fulminant CDC, which failed to improve on medical treatment. But whether a subtotal colectomy is advisable during an exploratory laparotomy in a critically ill patient for an acute abdomen, with a surprise operative finding of an undiagnosed CDC, is unknown. It appears that the construction of any bowel anastomosis is contra-indicated when operating on CDC – the ileum is exteriorized as an ileostomy and the rectum closed as a Hartmann's pouch.

21 Colonic Obstruction

The only time human beings wish they could defecate
and fart is when they are not able to do so

In this chapter we consider the most common cause of acute obstruction of the colon – *cancer*, but also mention a much less common cause which is *diverticulitis*. We'll have to discuss also the condition, which mimics obstruction – *pseudo-obstruction* or *Ogilvie's syndrome*. Finally, we'll deal with *volvulus of the colon*, that of the sigmoid and cecum.

Malignant and Diverticular Colonic Obstruction

The four "steps" you should consider in the approach to patients with mechanical colonic obstruction are:
- Establish the exact diagnosis and at operation:
- Decompress the colon.
- Resect the obstructing lesion.
- Decide whether there should be a primary anastomosis or a colostomy.

Preoperative Diagnosis and Management

The clinical hallmark of colonic obstruction is a significant abdominal distention associated with a recent onset of constipation and lack of flatus. The obstruction usually develops gradually over a few days, sometimes on a background of change in bowel habits. The usual site of the obstructing carcinoma is in the sigmoid or left colon. The sigmoid is also the locus of the obstructing diverticular mass. Right colonic lesion become ob-s}ructing only at the ileocecal region. Because of the wide caliber of the rectum – rectal cancer very rarely present with a complete obstruction.

Most of these patients are eleerly and because the obstruction may have affected them for several days, they have not been eating and drinking properly, leading to dehydration. Make a thorough examination of the abdomen. It is sometimes grossly distended but not all the time. Be especially observant about signs of peritonitis, which may indicate a manifest or pending perforation of the colon – usually proximal to the obstructing lesion. The site of perforation may be a pre-existing sigmoid or left colonic diverticulum but more commonly it is in the right colon. The right colon and cecum is the widest part of the bowel. It will also be the most distended part with the highest tension of the bowel wall (Laplace's law). When the ileocecal valve is competent the small bowel will be only mildly distended while massive distension and pressure affects the right colon. This pressure can tear the circular muscle layer or cause ischemic necrosis with subsequent perforation. Tenderness of the abdomen on the right side may be a sign of this development. If such tenderness is present and the abdominal X-ray show a grossly distended right colon (in excess of 10 cm) then the operation must not be delayed beyond the requirements of the resuscitation.

Plain abdominal X-rays (chapter 3) usually show a distended colon because the obstructing lesion is most often in the left colon. When the obstruction is in the right colon, at the cecal area, it can be sometimes difficult to differentiate between small bowel and large bowel obstruction. With long-standing left colonic obstruction, when the ileocecal valve is incompetent, the small bowel becomes dilated as well. Severely dilated loops of small bowel, and filled with fluid, may then obscure the distended colon – a picture which may be misinterpreted as a partial small bowel obstruction. Whatever you see on plain X-rays you have to confirm the diagnosis and exclude pseudo-obstruction (see below). Basically what you have to do is to document the site of the obstruction: this can be done either with fibro-optic *colonoscopy or a contrast enema*. For reasons explained in chapter 3 our bias is against the use of barium in this situation and in favor of a water-soluble contrast such as Gastrografin. The

site of the obstruction but not the cause will usually be evident. At this
stage 'obstruction is obstruction' – the management is the same whether
a carcinoma (common) or a diverticular mass (rare) causes it. A pre-
operative *CT scan* is not mandatory but may be useful in selective cases.
When clinical and laboratory features are suggestive of carcinomatosis,
or extensive hepatic metastatic involvement, CT documentation of the
advanced disease may allow a better planning of treatment together with
the patient and family. You do not want to operate on a jaundiced patient
whose liver is almost replaced with metastases for he'll surely succumb
to hepatic failure after the operation.

Planning and Timing the Operation

In general, in the absence of signs of actual or impending compromise of
the bowel wall there is no reason for you to hurry with the operation.
Daytime surgery, with all that it means in terms of the surgical team and
supportive personnel, is the better option for the patient and yourself. If
so, there is plenty time to prepare the patient for a definitive operation
to relieve the obstruction. On the other hand, should the patient have
peritonitis, SIRS, or free abdominal gas on the X-rays, an emergency
operation is necessary. Antibiotic treatment should be started and the
time of the operation decided according to the progress of the resuscitation – optimization (chapter 5).

Obviously, in patients with colonic obstruction bowel preparation
is contra-indicated. Any cleansing solutions administrated from above will
accumulate proximal to the obstruction – further dilating the obstructed
colon and making your life more miserable during the operation. Some
surgeons like to administer enemas to clear the rectum and colon distal
to the obstruction but these sections of the bowel are usually empty. Do
not forget to administer, just before the operation, the usual dose of
systemic antibiotic prophylaxis (chapter 6).

In general, the operation for acute colonic obstruction is a major procedure, often in a patient who is old and fragile. Consequently – the mortality and morbidity of these operations is significant (sorry – no percentages in this book). To avoid complications and mortality you have to exercise your best judgement according to the lines presented below.

The Operation

A long midline incision is nearly always preferable. The findings of ascites, peritoneal seedlings, "omental cake", and hepatic metastases will immediately tell you that the battle has been lost and the operation is merely palliative. If the obstruction is in the right colon there is usually not a lot of bowel distension. Then, the operation is rather straightforward as a right hemicolectomy with primary anastomosis. The left colon or the sigmoid, however, is the usual site of the obstruction. Here the proximal colon is distended making the operation more difficult. First inspect the ascending colon to find out if there are tears or necrosis due to the distension. If there are, they can be of any stage from minor to large with micro-perforation. The significance of the tears is that if they are extensive or necrotic it may suggest that a *subtotal colectomy* is indicated. Thus, proceed as follows:

- *Decompression*: Because of the distended bowel it may be difficult to expose the lesion on the left side and to manipulate the bowel. Sometimes it is better to make an enterotomy into the terminal ileum and insert the suction devise through the hole to decompress the small bowel and also pass the device through the ileocaecal valve to decompress the right colon. Close the hole with a suture. It should now be possible to expose the lesion that causes the obstruction. Often, in early diagnosed and treated cases, the colonic distention is caused by air and not fecal matter; it can be simply relieved by inserting a large needle or angiocath – connected to the suction tube – and tunneled through the tenia coil.

- *Resection*: Whether it is cancer or diverticulitis-sigmoiditis (chapter 23) the principles of treatment are the same. Mobilize the lesion the same way you would at an elective operation and resect it. If you are accustomed to linear cutting staplers (TLC or GIA) this is one of the best instances to use staplers. Transect the bowel on each side of the lesion and divide also the mesentery and the segmental vessels with the linear stapler. You have resected the cause of the obstruction with complete control of the bowel ends and no leakage. Now is the time to decide if the bowel ends should be joined or the proximal end should be brought out as a colostomy.

To Anastomose or Not?

The judgement process here is not much different from that considered after sigmoidectomy for acute diverticulitis as is discussed in chapter 23. What is different, however, is that here there is no associated peritonitis and suppuration. In essence after you resected the lesion you are left with a few options:

- End left (iliac) colostomy – Hartmann's procedure
- Primary colocolic or colorectal anastomosis
- Subtotal colectomy with ileosigmoid anastomosis

Do notice that it is considerably more difficult to operate on colonic obstruction than on a similar elective case. You will need the extra hands of an assistant to achieve exposure and the decisions are much more complex during the operation. It is advisable to do the operation together with a colleague who can assist with the decisions. If it is a cancer operation it should be the correct cancer resection not just an operation that relieves the obstruction. A "simple" bowel resection is permissible only if the cancer is disseminated so the type of resection has no influence on the prognosis of the cancer. In that situation a colostomy is usually the better option because it is safer for the patient and has less risk of a new obstruction due to the local recurrence of the tumor.

184   If the cancer is situated in the *transverse or descending colon* it is often better to do a *subtotal colectomy and an ileosigmoid anastomosis.* This usually means that empty or mildly distended and well-perfused small bowel is joined to normal colon below the obstruction. For cancers of the *sigmoid colon or rectosigmoid junction* a *sigmoid colectomy* is adequate and a subtotal colectomy should be considered only if the ascending colon is ischemic or perforated as mentioned above. Most patients will manage an ileosigmoid anastomosis without incapacitating diarrhea and incontinence, while an ileorectal anastomosis requires that the patient has had normal continence before the current illness.

The Colostomy

It should be understood that the creation of an emergency colostomy is potentially "problematic". A common problem is retraction due to inadequate mobilization of the bowel. It frequently causes disruption of the mucocutaneous suture line in the early postoperative course, followed by retraction of the bowel end to a subcutaneous position and progressive stenosis of the skin orifice. Even a retraction into the peritoneal cavity – resulting in peritoneal soiling with feces occasionally may occur. To be safe, make sure that the left colon has been mobilized up to the splenic flexure and sometimes including the left flexure. The closed proximal end should easily reach out several centimeters above skin level. Do not settle with anything less or you may make the patient´s remaining life an ordeal. The colostomy hole through the abdominis rectus muscle will have to be larger than normal because of the bowel distension. It is sometimes necessary to evacuate some of the gas and feces before the bowel can be brought out. A simple rule of thumb is that when the colostomy hole is distended with retractors the bowel end should pass "easily" between them, and it will not pass if the retractors are removed. There is no need to close the lateral gutter, or even to fixate the bowel to the anterior abdominal wall if it has been sufficiently mobilized.

The mucocutaneous suture of the colon to the skin with an absorbable
suture is all that is needed.

You should chose either an anastomosis or a colostomy. The proximal
"protective" 'ostomy for an anastomosis is a hybrid of a disputable value.
Should the anastomosis break, the "protective" colostomy is of little help
because the colon was not clean and will leak all the residual feces distal
to the protective stoma. A re-operation becomes necessary anyway. There
is no study that proves that the 'ostomy prevents the anastomotic failure.

Some Controversies

The main dispute is the primary anastomosis and the means of obtaining
that goal. It is only a problem for left-sided obstructions. *On-table bowel
irrigation* has been proposed to facilitate primary anastomosis between
clean proximal colon and the rectum. It value is discussed in chapter 23
on diverticulitis (section on *fecology*). The irrigation prolongs the operation substantially and therefore represents a "negative damage control".
An alternative is the *subtotal or total abdominal colectomy with anastomosis
of the terminal ileum to the sigmoid colon or rectum.* This also is a bigger
operation that takes longer time. In a large Scottish randomized trial
comparing the two means of obtaining a primary anastomosis there was
no difference in survival or anastomotic healing with either method.
There are now several randomized trials of elective colonic resection with
or without mechanical bowel preparation. Again there was no difference
in anastomotic healing. It may not be entirely valid to extrapolate the
results with residual feces of the "elective" colon to the massive fecal load
of the acute colon. It appears, however, that a primary anastomosis can
be made safely also on the obstructed colon after decompression and
removal of feces with suction and milking the colonic end before joining
it to the rectum. We, among others, make an anastomosis in an "unprepared bowel" in selective cases.

186   Why bother with a primary anastomosis at all when it increases the operation time and complexity of the operation? A Hartmann resection and colostomy is quicker and simpler. It is not an all or nothing situation but the concerned surgeon will know that the Hartmann resection is often the better choice if the patient is in bad general condition or if the cancer cannot be radically removed. About half of the Hartman resections will never be reversed, often for very good reasons. For the less experienced surgeon we would suggest that the Hartmann resection is always a valid option.

Is there any role for a decompressive colostomy without the resection of the obstructing lesion? This staged management was commonly used only a few decades ago, usually consisting of a transverse colostomy which represented the first stage. Nowadays we would reserve this option in two circumstances:

- The critically ill patient who won't tolerate a major procedure; for example – a patient developing an obstruction a week after a myocardial infarction. Here, a transverse colostomy or even cecostomy under local anesthesia will alleviate the obstruction.
- When there is pre-operative evidence of wide-spread malignant disease as discussed above.

Our own preferences: we believe that nowadays in most patients the resection of the obstructing lesion and a primary anastomosis can and should be achieved safely. For sigmoid lesions we would opt for a sigmoidectomy followed with a colorectal anastomosis; if the proximal colon is excessively "loaded" or appears "compromised" we would proceed with a subtotal colectomy and an ileorectal anastomosis. The latter is also our preference for lesions in the proximal descending colon and the transverse colon. We would reserve the Hartmann procedure to the "high risk patients" and those who appear poorly nourished.

Acute Colonic Pseudo-obstruction (Ogilvie's Syndrome)

This is an important differential diagnosis of mechanical colonic obstruction. The pseudo-obstruction has the same symptoms, signs, and radiographic appearances of acute large bowel obstruction but there is no mechanical blockage. The X-ray films suggest a left colon obstruction but a contrast study or colonoscopy finds no obstruction. The pseudo-obstruction can be so intense that the right colon becomes ischemic and perforates due to the high intra-mural pressure.

The mechanisms behind the pseudo-obstruction are not known. It has been proposed that the condition be due to sympathetic over-activity, parasympathetic suppression, or both. Most patients are already in hospital for other reasons when the pseudo-obstruction develops. It is a rare but well-recognized sequel to giving birth, but more commonly seen after major non-intestinal surgery or trauma, or on the background of serious medical illnesses.

This entity is the reason why you should not operate on a suspected colonic obstruction without a pre-operative contrast enema or colonoscopy. Taking an elderly patient with multiple pre-morbid conditions for a laparotomy to find "only" a distended colon, without an obstructing lesion, is a recipe for disaster. Avoid it! Instead, these patients should not be operated but be treated medically or decompressed wth colonoscopy. For the medical treatment it is suggested that Neostigmin (2 mg) effectively induces bowel movements and colonic emptying within a few minutes. There are side effects to the Neostigmin, including bradycardia, salivation, nausea and abdominal cramps. The patient should therefore be under close surveillance during the treatment. If medical treatment is ineffective, a colonoscopy may decompress the bowel. The target is decompression of the grossly distended cecum; occasionally, repeated colonoscopic decompressions may be needed. A large and long rectal tube can be left in situ after the colonoscopy for a few days. The diagnostic Gastrografin enema may occasionally be also therapeutic – the hyperosmolar contrast medium promoting colonic peristalsis (chapter 3).

Surgical treatment is required if the cecum perforates or very rarefy if medical treatment fails and the cecum reaches gigantic size. If the cecum becomes necrotic or perforates a right hemicolectomy is necessary. Because the functional obstruction must be in the left colon a primary anastomosis is inappropriate. It is better to fashion an end ileostomy and bring out the distal end of the colon through the same colostomy hole – fashioning a "double barrel" stoma. This arrangement makes it easy to later restore bowel continuity at the site of the colostomy without the need to re-open the abdomen. When at laparotomy the cecum is distended but viable most surgeons would opt for a cecostomy. Tube cecostomy is "messy"; it is associated with a high incidence of local complications such as a fecal leak around it or even into the abdomen. Use a large-bore and soft tube and surround it insertion site in the cecum with a double purse-string suture; the cecostomy site should be then carefully attached to the abdominal wall (as you do with a gastrostomy). Cecostomy tubes tend to obstruct with fecal matter and need regular flushing. A viable alternative to tube cecostomy is the "formal – matured cecostomy": simply exteriorize a portion of the cecum above the skin level and suture it to the surrounding skin. This, in the medically ill patients with pseudo-obstruction, can be easily performed under local anesthesia.

Volvulus of the Colon

While volvulus accounts for only one tenth of all instances of colonic obstruction we tend to remember those patients. It is probably because of the spectacular appearance on abdominal X-rays and the equally spectacular way it is treated. Volvulus of the sigmoid colon is by far the

most common, followed by that the cecum. There is also volvulus of the
transverse colon but it is so rare that you will probably not see even a
case during your surgical life.

Sigmoid Volvulus

In affected patients the sigmoid is long, with a redundant mesentery that
allows the sigmoid to rotate around its mesenteric axis, usually counter-
clockwise. We do not known why it occurs usually after patients have
reached seniority. It does happen in younger ages but then typically in
an institutionalized patient. The rotation must be at least 180 degrees to
be symptomatic for obstruction, but if the rotation is 360 degrees there
is also a risk of strangulation. These circumstances account for two types
of volvulus; a "slow" form where obstruction is progressively developing
and a "rapid" form where strangulation dominates. As the obstructing
point is distally at the recto-sigmoid junction – the propulsion of the
proximal colon will blow up the obstructed sigmoid loop to impressive
dimensions.

The typical patient presents with a history of recent onset consti-
pations and lack of flatus and grossly distended belly. Because half of the
patients have recurrent episodes of volvulus the diagnosis may already be
known. A plain abdominal film will suggest the diagnosis: a tremendously
large loop of colon fills the abdomen from the pelvis to the upper abdomen.
A contrast enema with gastrografin will show the obstruction at the
recto-sigmoid junction. Typically, the contrast ends in a "beak of-a-bird"
sign that is very characteristic. It is the lower twist that causes this image.

Treatment of Sigmoid Volvulus
Non-operative Approach
Until around 1950 the treatment of sigmoid volvulus was essentially
surgical and associated with a significant mortality. Then it was demonstrated that the volvulus could be decompressed with much lower M & M

190   by passing a tube through the rectum. There are three ways of doing the procedure. If you are lucky to work in a hospital where the radiologist treats the patient this is what they do. A large-bore flexible but rather stiff-size 30–36 and 50 cm long tube is passed through the anus and rectum to the site of obstruction. A bag of barium is connected to the tube and by letting in a little contrast the hydrostatic pressure will open the twisted bowel sufficiently to pass the tube into the obstructed sigmoid. A flush of gas and feces signifies the successful decompression. The whole procedure is done under X-ray imaging. Whether the tube should be left in place for a day or withdrawn immediately is a matter of debate.

You might have to do the procedure yourself without the assistance of imaging. Then, use a rigid rectoscope and pass it to the twist, which should be seen. The lubricated tube is introduced through the rectoscope and carefully manipulated into the sigmoid. A third method is by means of a flexible colonoscopy and maneuvering the scope itself into the sigmoid. The eventual success of your manipulations is usually announced with a sudden rush of flatus and fecal matter at your face.

Operative Treatment

The non-operative methods are successful in the vast majority of cases because strangulation is uncommon. If strangulation and necrosis of the sigmoid is suspected on clinical grounds (evidence of peritonitis) or if attempts at non-operative decompression fail, then an emergency laparotomy is required. At operation (lithotomy position) you will encounter a hugely distended sigmoid colon which has to be decompressed. This is best achieved by gently untwisting the sigmoid and advancing a pre-positioned rectal tube into the dilated segment. Today, in most patients who undergo an emergency operation for sigmoid volvulus the bowel will be non-viable or compromised. Thus, the procedure of choice is sigmoid resection – either with a colorectal anastomosis or as a Hartmann's procedure. The selection of what to do is essentially the same as discussed

above with regard to malignant colonic obstruction. Finally, we have to
mention the option of sigmoidopexy – the fixation of the sigmoid to the
lateral abdominal wall. This is a theoretical option when the sigmoid is
viable, and well decompressed, and you think that sigmoid resection
with anastomosis is "too much" for the individual patient.

After a Successful Non-operative Decompression

The elective sigmoidectomy to prevent recurrence, on the other hand, is
very simple. It is done with a small transverse incision through which
the hypertrophied mobile sigmoid loop is delivered and resected. There
is no general agreement when patients should be offered a sigmoidectomy to prevent a recurrence. About half of the patients will have only one
episode but those with two episodes will frequently have a third. Most
surgeons therefore offer resection after the second episode. Anecdotally,
a fragile lady in her mid 80's suffered one episode after the other but
each time she was thought unfit for an elective operation of a benign
condition. After her twelfth volvulus she had proved her case and was
subjected to sigmoidectomy from which she recovered uneventfully and
was discharged after five days.

Volvulus of the Cecum

This is much less common – you'll probably won't see more than 4 cases
during your career – but will usually require an operation. The diagnosis
is not as straightforward as that of the sigmoid volvulus. These patients
have clinical and radiographic signs of small bowel obstruction. In
addition, typically, the cecal "shadow" is absent from the right lower
quadrant. Instead, the poorly attached and redundant cecum, which has
flipped to the left and upwards, is visualized in the epigastrium or the
left hypochondrium – with its concavity pointing to the right lower
quadrant. A single fluid level may be seen – representing the dislocated
cecum and often confused with the gastric shadow. If in doubt, and in

the absence of peritoneal signs, order a Gastrografin enema, which will demonstrated the characteristic "beak" in the right colon.

There are isolated reports of colonoscopic decompression of cecal volvulus but the complexity of such procedure and its doubtful results suggest that operation is the treatment of choice. What to do? There is an eternal controversy – probably never to be solved – between the proponents of cecal fixation-cecopexy, and the advocates of mandatory resection. This is our selective approach: first de-tort the cecum; the torsion is clockwise so de-rotate the mobile cecum. If after de-torsion the bowel appears gangrenous or of doubtful viability – roceed with a right hemi-colectomy. A primary anastomosis should be usually permissible but occasionally circumstances suggest that an ostomy is preferable. If so, bring out the small bowel as an end ileostomy and a corner of the closed colon's end through the same ostomy hole. This combined "double-barrel" ostomy allows simple closure and restoration of bowel continuity through the site of the ostomy.

If it the cecum is viable we see no point is resecting it. Why remove a healthy organ which can be "fixed"? To prevent recurrence of the volvulus, fix the mobile cecum to the lateral abdominal wall-i.e. cecopexy. Start with the decompression of the cecum, by "milking" it towards a rectal tube, for sutures hold poorly in a distended bowel wall. Cecopexy is accomplished by suturing the entire length of the cecum to the lateral abdominal wall. Use non-absorbable material and take big seromuscular bites on the bowel and big-deep bites on the abdominal side. Some surgeons elevate a flap of parietal peritoneum that is sutured to the anterior wall of the cecum.

Cecostomy, either a tube or 'matured' to the skin, is an option, which is mentioned in the literature as an alternative to cecopexy. We however think that it is a bad idea: why convert a simple and clean procedure (i.e. cecopexy) to a contaminated and potentially complicated one (i.e. cecostomy)?

22 Acute Appendicitis

Whatever is the clinical presentation,
whichever are the abdominal findings,
always consider acute appendicitis at the back of your mind.

Acute appendicitis (AA) is discussed in any surgical text dating from the turn of the 19th century. Looking at the lengthy chapters devoted to this subject we often wonder what is there to chat so much about. Knowing that you were fed on AA ad nauseum since the early days of medical school we do not intend to repeat here the whole 'spiel' again. Instead, we promise to be brief and not to bore.

Diagnosis

AA is an inflammation – turning into infection – of the appendix. This rudimentary structure varies in length and position, making matters complicated. Even a dentist (but not a gynecologist) can diagnose a case of 'classical' AA: the history of mid-abdominal, 'visceral' pain, shifting to the right lower quadrant (RLQ) and becoming 'somatic' – localized speaks for itself. Add to it the clinical and laboratory evidence of systemic inflammation/infection and, most essential, the localized physical findings of peritoneal irritation. Unfortunately or fortunately (otherwise dentists will be treating AA) for each 'classical' case you will see two 'atypical' cases. Sure, you know by now that AA is missed at the extremes of age, that in menstruating females it is often confused with gynecological conditions (chapter 25), that retrocecal and pelvic appendices are probably more problematic, and that it should be 'always on your mind' – at least 'number two' on your list of differential diagnosis. So what can we add that you do not know? Probably nothing. But let us emphasize a few points:

194 • Never confirm or exclude the diagnosis of AA on the presence or absence of one or more symptom, sign or finding "that must be there" as such an obligatory variable does not exist. Instead, suspect AA from the synthesis of the whole clinical picture and constellation of the various variables.

• Every budding surgeon feels compelled to design his own "screening test" for AA. The "cough test", the "jump sign" the "please bring your tummy to my finger test" and many others. They are all fun but none approaches the sensitivity or specificity of 90 per cent (oops, sorry, we promised not to use percentages). The truth is that the accuracy of the clinical diagnosis of AA cannot be perfect. Should your policy to operate be based only on clinical assessment and basic laboratory values – a reasonable approach – then one to two out of ten of the appendixes removed will be normal-white'. More than that implies that you are a 'cowboy'; less would suggest that you are dangerously prudent.

So you seriously suspect AA after having excluded, or at least you believe so, a gynecological or urological pathology, gastroenteritis, mesenteric lymphadenitis, or the trash bin called "nonspecific abdominal pain". Should you now proceed directly to the operating theatre or order imaging modalities?

Abdominal Imaging in Acute Appendicitis

The "diagnostic" finding of non-filling appendix on *barium enema* was previously quoted by radiologists trying to convince us to load the patient's colon with barium in order to diagnose AA. As emphasized previously, the use of barium in emergency surgery is a recipe for disasters and anyway, the idea of enema did not catch on. *Ultrasound* in 'good

hands' has been reported to be accurate in the diagnosis of AA and may
be useful to exclude other diagnoses, which may require different therapy
(e.g. hydronephrosis) or incision (e.g. acute cholecystitis). Also *CT* may
demonstrate the peri-cecal inflammatory changes and associated fluid
collections of AA. *Fine needle aspiration* of the peritoneum for cytological
examination has been reported as extremely exact. But should we waste
money and time and obtain additional testing? We do not think so. *We
would order imaging selectively.* For example, when an "appendiceal
mass" is suspected or when exclusion of other non-operatively treated
condition is crucial (e.g. neutropenic entrocolitis in the immunocompro-
mised patient or abdominal pain complex in AIDS).

What about *laparoscopic diagnosis*? It is of particular value in the
young female – to exclude and treat gynecological conditions, avoiding
the open appendectomy scar (chapter 25). Obviously, should you be one
of those thinking that 'everything is better with the laparoscope' you
could start any operation with a diagnostic laparoscopy, and then proceed. More on this issue read in chapter 41.

Periodic re-evaluation: before moving on to treatment we wish to
mention that the best diagnostic modality in the doubtful case is *watchful
waiting*. Unfortunately, the art of periodic re-examinations and the virtue
of patience are disappearing from the scene of modern practice where
the emphasis is on obsessive activity, when in order to prove oneself –
one has always to "do something". In the absence of clear peritonitis and
toxicity, very rarely are attacks of AA a true emergency requiring an
immediate operation. If undecided, admit the patient and periodically
re-examine him or her over the day or night. In most instances, the AA
will declare itself and, if it is not AA, the "attack" will resolve. *Note:* if you
decide to observe the patient, do not administer antibiotics as it may
mask the findings, "partially treat", or even cure the AA.

Classification

Let us bring here a simple classification of AA to facilitate the discussion of management. Basically, AA is either *"simple"* or *"complicated"*. "Simple" AA implies inflammation of the appendix of any extent in *the absence of appendiceal gangrene, perforation or peri-appendicular pus formation.* Define AA as "complicated" whenever any of the aforementioned is present.

Another term you should be familiar with is the *appendiceal mass*, developing late in the natural history of AA. The "mass" is an inflammatory phlegmon made of omentum or/adjacent viscera, walling off a "complicated" appendix. A "mass" containing a variable amount of pus is an *appendiceal abscess*.

Management

Antibiotics

Judicious administration of antibiotics, possessing *anti-gram negative and anaerobes* spectrum, will minimize the incidence of postoperative wound (common) and intra-abdominal (rare) infective complications. in "simple" AA the antibiotics are considered *prophylactic*, while in "complicated" AA they are *therapeutic*. We encourage you to administer the first dose of antibiotics pre-operatively just before you scrub. If at surgery the AA prove to be "simple", no postoperative administration is necessary. Should you, on the other hand, discover "complicated" AA, additional postoperative doses are indicated. We suggest that you tailor the duration of administration to the operative findings. Gangrenous AA, without any pus formation, represent a "resectable infection" which does not require more than 24 hours of postoperative administration. Perforated AA with or without intra-peritoneal pus should be treated longer but *for no more than 5 days.* (chapters 6,10 & 32)

Perhaps you are not aware that most attacks of "simple" AA would
respond to non-operative management with antibiotics. Also "complicated"
AA may respond to antibiotics or at least could "mature" into an abscess.
So why don't we treat most cases of AA initially conservatively, along the
same lines as acute diverticulitis (chapter 23) of the sigmoid colon?
Because surgical management of AA is simpler and less morbid than
that of diverticulitis. When faced with AA away from surgical facilities
(e.g. at mid ocean) you should treat the patient with antibiotics (which
should be available on any ship). Also the preferred management of an
"appendiceal mass" is conservative as discussed below.

Operation

When to Operate?

Not with each patient diagnosed as AA you have to rush to the operating
room ASAP! Obviously if your patient is systemically "sick" and his
abdominal findings are impressive (denoting a perforation) – operate
immediately. Otherwise, a few hours of delay, while the patient receives
antibiotics are acceptable. You do not rush to the OR with acute diverticulitis (chapter 23); so what's the difference?

Only the "open" procedure will be discussed, as the evidence
hitherto does not support the notion that laparoscopic appendectomy is
advantageous. The special value of laparoscopy in the difficult to diagnose
female patient is mentioned in chapter 25; a morbidly obese patient may
be another relative indication. Should you like, however, to play with gas,
sticks and staplers help yourself! For more about this controversy see
chapter 41.

We are convinced that you have done your share of appendectomies
already as an intern. Having seen, however, many surgeons who transform
a customary appendectomy to an elaborate operation resembling a
Whipple's procedure, we will advise you to KISS (keep it simple stupid-
schmuck).

- *Incision*: you do not need the long unsightly oblique incision. Use the transverse one. A common error is to place it too medially over the rectus sheath; stay lateral to it. Start with a mini-incision; it can be always enlarged.
- *Appendectomy*: you can remove the appendix in an antegrade or retrogarde fashion but there is no need to invert the stump – unless you are hooked on useless rituals. So just ligate or suture-transfix the appendix at its base and chop the rest off. The commonly performed rituals of "painting" the stump with Betadine or "burning" it with diathermy are simply ridiculous.
- *Peritoneal toilet*: just suck out the fluid and few drops of pus, which float around, and mop it up with a dry gauze-stick (do not forget the pelvis). Do not perform peritoneal lavage through this keyhole incision. It is unnecessary and useless.
- *Drains*: almost never necessary and may be indicated (perhaps) only after the drainage of a large appendicular abscess. Never exit the drains through the main incision.
- *Closure*: separate closure of the peritoneum is not necessary. Instillation of an antibiotic in the fat – protects against wound infection (in addition to the systemic administration). Do not insert subcutaneous sutures (foreign bodies). Our bias is for primary closure of the skin in all cases. A few will develop wound infection managed by removal of (a few) stitches. Isn't it better than secondary closure, which condemns all patients to further manipulations and an ugly scar? (chapters 29 & 40)

The "White" Appendix

What should you do when the appendix proves to be normal-"white"?
Well, you can "rub" it to allow the pathologist to diagnose mild acute
inflammation (just kidding). The classical dictum is that whenever an
abdominal appendectomy incision exists the appendix should be removed
in order not to confuse matters in the future. What about a normal appendix visualized at laparoscopy? Should it be also removed? The emerging
consensus is to leave it alone, informing the patient or his parents that
the appendix has been left in situ. But this remains controversial.

Obviously, when the appendix appears normal you should search
for alternative diagnoses such as Meckel's diverticulitis, adnexal pathology,
or mesenteric lymphadenitis. In most instances, however, you'll find
nothing. What should you do if foul smelling, murky, or bile-stained
peritoneal fluid is encountered, suggesting serious alternate pathology
elsewhere? Bile should guide you into the upper abdomen. Close the
incision and place a new one where "the action is". Feces or its odor direct
you towards the sigmoid; just extent the incision across the midline and
you are there. *No incision signifies an indecision, provided you can decide.*

The "Valentino Appdenix"

Intra-peritoneal inflammation from any cause can inflame-inject the
appendix from the "outside" – mimicking AA. This was the case with the
famous movie actor and womanizer Rudolph Valentino who underwent
an appendectomy for suspected acute appendicitis in New York (1926).
He became gravely ill after the operation and died; autopsy revealed a
perforated peptic ulcer. The findings of peritoneal fluid and suppuration,
together with a "mildly inflamed" and non-gangrenous and non- perforated
appendix should raise your suspicion that the pathology is elsewhere –
look for it!

200   The Post-appendectomy Appendiceal Stump Phlegmon

Your patient had an uneventful appendectomy for acute appendicitis following which he happily went home. Seven days later he presents with a left lower quadrant pain, temperature and high white cell count. The operative site looks OK. This is a typical presentation of an appendix stump phlegmon. Nowadays the diagnosis is simple: a CT will demonstrate a phlegmon, which involves the cecum – as opposed to a drainable abscess. A few days of antibiotic therapy will cure this relatively rare complication, which for some reasons is not mentioned by "standard texts".

Appendiceal Mass

Typically, patients with an appendiceal mass present late in the course of the disease, with symptoms of an 'abdominal condition' lasting a week or more. Occasionally, they report a spontaneous improvement in their symptoms, reflecting the localization of the inflammatory process. On clinical examination you will find a right iliac fossa mass. Overlying tenderness or obesity may obscure the presence of the mass. Therefore, suspect an appendiceal mass in the 'late presenters' or those with an atypical 'smoldering' picture. When palpation is not rewarding, obtain a CT scan, which is the best diagnostic modality to document the appendiceal mass. Another indication for the CT is associated evidence of undrained pus such a spiking fever and toxicity, signifying an *appendiceal abscess*.

Why should you distinguish between AA and appendiceal mass (or abscess) if the management of these conditions is the same (i.e. operation and antibiotics)? *Because the appendiceal mass (and abscess) can be managed non-operatively.* You could operate on both, as you operate on

AA, but the removal of the appendix involved in an inflammatory mass
may be more hazardous than usual, occasionally necessitating as "much"
as a right hemicolectomy. On the other hand, conservative treatment
with antibiotics leads to the resolution of the mass in the vast majority
of cases. As no more than one out of five patients will suffer a recurrence
of AA (usually within 1 year and not a severe attack) the dogma of
routine 'interval appendectomy' within 6 weeks has become obsolete.
Interestingly, in many of these patients during 'interval appendectomy'
the appendix is rudimentary-scarred. In patients over the age of 40 years
we suggest an elective colonoscopy and CT scan (after 3 months) to
exclude the rare situation in which cecal carcinoma was the cause of the
mass.

Failure of the mass to respond to antibiotics signifies an abscess.
CT or ultrasound guided percutaneous drainage is the most rational
approach (chapter 35). Failure to clinically improve within 48 hours
means that operation is needed. At operation drain the pus and remove
the appendix if it is "not too difficult".

With a high index of suspicion you can obviate an operation in the
majority of patients with an appendiceal mass. *And, remember: appendiceal
mass represents an unfavorable situation for your laparoscopic skills.*

Appendicitis Epiploica

We mention this condition here because of its name, because you probably
did not hear much about it, and because it is not so rare and often
imitates AA. Appendicitis epiploica follows a spontaneous torsion of the
appendix epiploica – the peritoneum-covered tabs of fat attached along
the tenia of colon. It is more common in obese individuals and in the
cecum and sigmoid. Since the sigmoid colon often crosses the midline
the most common manifestation is localized tenderness and 'peritoneal
signs' in the right iliac fossa. Typically, patients do not feel or appear

202   'sick' despite these findings. Thus, "AA on examination" in an afebrile and healthy looking patient should rise your suspicion. The natural history is spontaneous remission as the appendix epiploica sloughs off, transforming into a "loose calcified peritoneal body". CT scan may identify the localized area of peri-colonic inflammation. If you are misled into an operation just remove the necrotic piece of fat.

Conclusions

Like any other surgical condition, acute appendicitis has a *spectrum*. To arrive at the diagnosis, consider together historical, physical and laboratory variables. No isolated variable can confirm or exclude AA, while the more "typical" variables are present, the higher is the chance that you are dealing with AA. Whether you operate immediately or tomorrow, whether you observe or obtain additional tests – is determined *selectively* based on your individual patient.

23 Acute Diverticulitis* 203

Think about acute diverticulitis as a left-sided acute appendicitis which is, however, usually treated without an operation"

Diverticula of the colon are not "true" diverticula but herniations of the mucosa through a weak spot of the muscular bowel wall. They can occur in all parts of the colon but are most abundant in the sigmoid colon. The mucosa bulges out through the points of entry for the blood vessels, which transgress the bowel wall on each side, where the mesentery joins the bowel. It is thought that the pressure inside the sigmoid colon, which can be very high, causes the expulsion of the mucosa. The smooth muscle of sigmoid colon, unlike that of the rest of the colon and rectum, is often hypertrophied. This thickening is always located at the summit of the sigmoid loop and rarely extends for more than 15 cm'. The diverticula mainly appear within this thickened segment of the sigmoid but are not restricted to it. It may develop at the rectosigmoid junction but never extend into the rectum proper (15 cm from anal verge). However, it is common to find diverticula extending into the descending colon. Be aware that *diverticulosis* – the mere presence of sigmoid diverticula is extremely prevalent in persons consuming a Western-type diet, while *acute diverticulitis* – inflammation of the diverticula-bearing segment of the colon – is relatively much rarer.

Surgical Pathology

A wide spectrum of pathological conditions is covered by the term of acute diverticulitis – each correlating with a specific clinical scenario which in turn necessitates selective management.

---

* At the end of this chapter you'll find also a few words on *perforation of the colon during colonoscopy.*

At operation for acute diverticulitis the sigmoid usually feels like a thick fusiform tumor, with only a few diverticula. There are also cases with minor thickening with many diverticula, one of which has perforated and is the cause of the acute inflammation. Such observations makes one think about the basic pathology of acute diverticulitis. Morson, the famous pathologist at St Marks', London, highlighted the hypertrophy of the bowel wall as the primary pathology and we are inclined to accept that, with the addition that the mesenteric fat tissue also plays a role. It is the fat that creeps up the bowel wall, becomes inflamed, produces the flegmon or abscess, and heals with fibrosis. In our experience, many cases of acute diverticulitis would rather be termed *acute sigmoiditis* – recognizing that it is an acute inflammation of the thickened bowel wall and mesentery. When it is a diverticulum that has been eroded by a fecalith, one finds a localized inflammation, which identifies the site of the perforation. In cases of free fecal peritonitis a perforated diverticulum is the cause although more often it has been walled off by the mesentery or epiploic appendices to produce a peri-colic abscess. Sometimes, the perforation occurs entirely within the mesentery, forming a mesenteric phlegmon or abscess. The latter may secondarily perforate into the free peritoneal cavity but usually this variety only gives rise to minor abdominal and systemic signs.

There is a strong tendency for diverticulitis and sigmoiditis to locally adhere and *fistulate*. The formation of fistula has an obscure mechanism as most patients with such fistula present as non-emergency cases and often do not even give a history of previous attacks of acute diverticulitis. Most often the fistula are into the bladder. The patient seeks attention for pneumaturia or persistent urinary tract infection. Fistula can also communicate with the Fallopian tubes, the uterus, small bowel or the skin. It is usually thought that the fistula is the sequel of an abscess but commonly there is no sign of an associate abscess; if there was one it must have been silent or drained spontaneously via the fistulous tract.

Clinical Features, Diagnosis and Approach   205

It is clinically pragmatic to think about acute diverticulitis or sigmoiditis as a "left-sided acute appendicitis". Unlike appendicitis, however, most episodes of acute diverticulitis are successfully managed without an operation. Practically, we find it convenient to think about the clinical scenarios of acute diverticulitis in order of increasing severity:

•   *Simple-phlegmonous diverticulitis*
COMPLICATED FORMS
•   Peri-colic abscess
•   Free perforation with purulent peritonitis
•   Free perforation with fecal peritonitis

Phlegmonous Diverticulitis

Most patients admitted to the hospital with acute diverticulitis harbor a phlegmon: they are still capable of mounting an anti-inflammatory response that quenches the inflammation. Such patients are in good condition but suffer from acute pain and tenderness in the left lower quadrant and above the symphysis pubis. A mass may be felt on abdominal or rectal examination. There are signs of systemic inflammation with fever, leukocytosis with left shift. For this stage the diagnosis is clinical. The patient is treated conservatively and usually responds.

Conservative Treatment of Acute Diverticulitis

Traditionally patients with "mild"-phlegmonous diverticulitis are admitted to the hospital; they are kept nil per mouth and on IV fluids. Wide spectrum antibiotics are given and continued until local and systemic inflammatory manifestation subsides. The colon however contains feces and will contain feces even after a few days of starvation. So what is the rational of the "traditional" regimen? We contend that in the absence of an associated intestinal ileus you may feed your patient or at least provide him with oral fluids instead of the IV. The same is also true concerning antibiotics: a perfectly adequate "coverage" of anaerobic and aerobic colonic bacteria can be achieved using oral agents such as metronidazole & 'cipro' (chapters 6, 10 & 32). So if IV therapy is not necessary – why admit the patient at all? And in fact mild acute diverticulitis can be managed with oral antibiotics on an outpatient basis.

Complicated Diverticulitis

In the minority of diverticulitis patients local and systemic signs of inflammation will persist or increase over the next couple of days. This is when you should start considering the presence of complicated forms of diverticulitis. Now it is time to order an abdominal CT (chapter 3) to better define the pathological anatomy. Ambrosetti in Geneva has devised criteria to grade acute diverticulitis on CT in a clinically meaningful way:

- *Simple attack*: bowel wall thickness of more than 5 mm with signs of inflammation of the pericolic fat.
- *Severe attack*: In addition: abscess, extra-luminal gas or leakage of contrast.

About half of the patients found on CT to have a "severe attack" required an operation during the current admission or subsequent to it. Significantly, however, half of such patients do *not* require an operation, suggesting that CT findings are to be used *together* with the clinical picture in tailoring the proper management.

Should you order a "routine" CT in all patients suspected to suffer from acute diverticulitis? This surely is an unnecessary "overkill" as

most patients respond to conservative treatment. In addition, in many
instances of clinically mild diverticulitis the CT is "negative".

Approach to Complicated Diverticulitis

A small number of patients present from the start with diffuse peritonitis;
with or without free intra-peritoneal air on AXR (chapter 2 & 3). Here of
course a CT scan is a waste of time better spent in the intensive care unit
for preoperative preparation (chapter 5). The final diagnosis will then be
established at the operation. The same applies for patients who show
signs of spreading peritonitis and increasing systemic inflammation
accompanied by tachycardia, tachypnea, hypovolemia with oliguria,
hypoxia or acidosis.

CT manifestations of a *"severe attack"* (i.e. extraluminal gas, leakage
of contrast or abscess) in a patient who failed to respond to a few days of
antibiotics are not an immediate indication for an operation. Instead, in
the want of spreading abdominal signs, or systemic deterioration, even
small (<5 cm') pericolic abscesses usually resolve without an operation
(probably spontaneously draining back into the bowel). In such cases we
would advice, therefore, to continue with conservative treatment.

Larger peri-colic *abscesses* (>5 cm') should be drained; this is best
done percutaneously under CT guidance. After the successful drainage a
"semi-elective" resection of the sigmoid is usually recommended. We do
not know, however, whether this is absolutely necessary. An unknown
percentage of such patients would probably never develop another attack
of acute diverticulitis.

The Operation for Acute Diverticulitis

When you are "forced" to operate for acute diverticulitis the procedure
of choice is sigmoidectomy. It is usually best to open the abdomen with

208   a lower midline incision, which should extend above the umbilicus to allow access to the descending colon, and be extended further to reach the left flexure should it be necessary to mobilize it. The inflamed sigmoid has frequently folded itself into the pelvis – adherent to the left pelvic brim, and may rest against the bladder or uterus. At times it will descend further into the pelvis between the rectum and bladder in the man and behind the uterus and upper vagina in the woman, depending upon how deep the fossa is. The differential diagnosis of a perforated cancer easily comes to mind. A clue is to remember that the inflammation is always at the summit of the sigmoid loop. The rectum and the rectosigmoid junction anterior to the promontory are always unaffected. It is usually possible to reach the anterior rectum from the right side of the pelvis to identify the folding of the sigmoid. Try not to use sharp dissections in this inflammatory and adherent situation; using finger dissection is your best bet; gentle finger-pinching and fracture will tear away fat and edema – leaving the vessels to be clamped and secured.

This is not a cancer operation and your aim basically is to remove the sigmoid colon, which is the source of the problem. Staying near the bowel wall helps you also to stay out of danger – away from the left ureter and ovarian vessels, which may be part of the inflammatory mass. It is best to start dividing the mesentery away from the inflammatory process below and above the sigmoid. After dividing and clamping (or using a linear stapler) the sigmoid at both ends – the rest of the sigmoid mesentery is dealt with. It is prudent to suture-liagte vessels within the thick-edematous mesentery rather then use simple ligatures that may slip. Using a vascular cartridge in a linear stapler to control the mesentery is another – albeit more expensive – alternative. Remove now any residual blood, pus or intestinal contents (chapter 10) and consider the next step.

To Anastomose or Not?

Should the two bowel ends be joined together or is a Hartmann procedure with an end sigmoid colostomy to be preferred? An anastomosis is justified in the majority of patients but there are a number of factors to consider. Localized peritonitis or an abscess are certainly not contraindications to an anastomosis. Generalized peritonitis is also not a contraindication in itself but the surgeon needs to give it a special consideration. Whether purulent or feculent the generalized peritonitis signifies a greater insult to the patient as reflected by the corresponding APACHE II score and the higher risk of dying (chapter 5). The operative trauma adds its share to the postoperative SIRS and MODS (chapter 38). Most patients with generalized peritonitis due to perforated diverticulitis have an immunology defect – not allowing localization of the process. Typically, they suffer from chronic obstructive lung disease or chronic arthritis with anti-inflammatory drugs or steroid dependence for years. Occasionally they received chemotherapy or are just recovering from major surgery such as a coronary bypass. On the other hand it seems that patients without such immunology defects are capable of containing the inflammation and rarely have free peritonitis. Patients with free peritonitis will certainly not tolerate an anastomotic failure and it is all the better if there is no need to worry about the integrity of an anastomosis during the postoperative course. Therefore, in such patients we chose a *Hartmann's procedure* – sigmoidectomy, end-colostomy and closing of the rectal stump.

It is our impression that surgeons pay little attention to the consequences of the operative trauma added to the acute inflammation. We find surgeons blaming the unfavorable course of some of these patients on the diverticulitis and peritonitis, believing that residual infection is the problem. They should instead consider the operative trauma and postoperative SIRS. If a sick patient is thrown out the window (inadvertently of course) and the surgeon then blames the subsequent

210   course on the illness we would all say it is a misconception of the situation. The height the patient falls is the operative trauma. The longer the operation takes, the more dissection that was necessary and the more bleeding it caused – the greater is the operative trauma. All this translates into a modern concept of damage control (chapters 10 & 27) and surgeons need to have a firm understanding of when enough is enough. If it is, the patient will have a worse course and an anastomosis may be inappropriate.

Fecology

Reasonable amounts of feces in the colon are not a contraindication for an anastomosis. You can evacuate most of the feces from the left colon by milking it into a dish. Occasionally, however, the colon may contain large amounts of fecal material because the sigmoiditis have caused a relative obstruction in the days preceding the acute attack. Massive fecal loading is a factor against an anastomosis. It has been proposed that on-table antegrade bowel irrigation (through the cecum or appendiceal stump) be added to clean the colon before the anastomosis. Unless such irrigation is common practice in your hospital, with all the equipment available, the irrigation will take at least an hour and often much more to accomplish. The subsequent anastomosis will add another 20 to 30 minutes to the operation. If this is the case an ostomy is quicker and gives a better damage control. In sum: consider an anastomosis in patients who are in a reasonable health and without diffuse peritonitis. There should be no technical problems to make the anastomosis if the bowel ends are healthy and without tension. How to do it – consult chapter 11.

A Few Controversies

- Some surgeons believe that the inflamed mesentery should be anatomically resected together with the sigmoid – claiming that it usually provides for a better anastomosis when there is no intervening mesentery left.
- Should the left flexure always be mobilized? No. This is indicated only in the minority of patients in whom the proximal colon fails to reach the rectum for a good anastomosis without tension, or in patients in whom the blood flow in the marginal artery is uncertain. Diverticula of the descending colon are common but we do not hesitate to anastomose diverticula-containing descending colon to the rectum. Recurrent diverticulitis proximal to the sigmoid is extremely rare.
- What should you do with phlegmonous diverticulitis, which is accidentally discovered during operation with no frank perforation or suppuration present? Probably do nothing at all; just close-up and treat with antibiotics. Most such patients will never return.

Newer Concepts

There are reports of successful laparoscopic management with peritoneal lavage of perforated diverticulitis and generalized peritonitis, without the resection of the involved bowel. All patients recovered uneventfully and were well during 12–24 months of follow-up. The concept that emerges is that the disease process can be reversed without a bowel resection, which can be postponed or not be performed at all. Larger experience is necessary to validate such an approach.

212   After the Attack

Most patients with acute diverticulitis respond to conservative therapy; it is estimated that around one-fourth will experience a recurrence. Somewhat confusingly this is variably interpreted as either confirming the need for elective surgery or indicating that the majority of patients do not require an operation. A second attack is probably an indication for an elective sigmoidectomy – this being particularly true in the younger patient.

Looking at the "whole picture" it appears that we operate too early in acute diverticulitis, perform too many CT's, carry out too many PC drainage procedures, remove too many colons, exteriorize too many colostomies, re-operate electively on too many patients, and perform too few randomized controlled trials in order to know what is right and what is wrong.

Perforation of the Colon During Colonoscopy

We elected to "insert" this topic at the end of the chapter which deals with diverticulitis because the approach to this situation is not dissimilar.

Instrumental perforation of the colon is not uncommon. How many such cases you will see depends on how busy are your local gastroenterological buddies. A specialty which bases its living on inserting large tubes from above and below is bound to provide you with a few such complications each year. In general, colonic perforations following colonoscopy occur through two main mechanisms, which are associated with distinct clinical presentations:

- Rupture of the colon due to over inflation combined with mechanical trauma caused by the scope itself. Here the perforation occurs during the procedure with the clinical signs evident immediately thereafter. Such traumatic ruptures are usually large and intra-peritoneal.

- Perforation of the colon at the site of a polypectomy. This may develop already during the procedure but more commonly "traumatic polypectomy" results in bowel wall-burn/necrosis, with the actual perforation developing within a day or two after the colonoscopy. Such perforations may be minute or develop initially within the leafs of the mesocolon, thenceforward invading the peritoneal cavity.

The following approach to iatrogenic colonic perforations is based on the specific clinical scenario, assisted by the selective use of radiological investigations. Such approach should save the vast majority of the affected patients although only during the two last years we had the opportunity to review the charts of two patients who died following colonoscopic perforations. In both – the colonoscopy was probably not indicated and the management of this complication faulty.

- Any abdominal pain after a colonoscopy should be taken seriously even if occurring a few days after the procedure as late perforation of necrotic areas or initially silent-contained perforations are not uncommon.
- The patient should be admitted and evaluated immediately as any "acute abdomen" (chapters 2 & 3). Clinical peritonitis is an indication for a laparotomy. You will always find a significant colonic "rent".
- Minimal, local abdominal findings plus scanty systemic repercussions suggest the possibility of a "mini" or "self-sealed" perforation. Here the patient can be treated selectively. Conservative treatment with antibiotic is often possible and effective provided that a "free" leak has been excluded with a gastrografin enema. Adding a CT to the contrast enema would allow picking up details such as the amount of free peritoneal fluid and local inflammatory changes.
- Localized abdominal findings with no evidence of free leak on gastrografin and/or CT allow you to continue with non-operative management. It will be successful in the majority of so treated cases.

214 •   On the other hand, non-contained leakage on abdominal imaging
        and/or worsening clinical picture will force you to operate.
        Following the above guidelines you'll intervene early enough
        before the 'contamination' has progressed to 'infection' (chapter 10)
        and anyway, usually the contamination is minimal because the
        colon has been prepared for colonoscopy. Therefore, at laparotomy
        primary repair of the bowel defect is almost always indicated and
        possible (no difference here from traumatic colonic perforations-
        chapter 27). Colostomy is very rarely indicated: in cases with
        neglected intra-abdominal infection or critical condition due to
        delayed diagnosis or underlying malnutrition (chapter 11).

**The mechanism of the perforation determines the size of the hole,
which should be thus managed selectively by the smart surgeon –
not the "blind" gastroeneterologist.**

24 Massive Rectal Bleeding

It's not bleeding until you can hear it bleeding
(Gail Waldby)

"Massive bleeding" is defined as 'exanguinating' and/or hemodynamically significant bleeding, which persists and requires 4 to 6 units of blood over a period of 24 hours. Fortunately, truly massive bleeding from the colon and rectum is unusual. The vast majority of episodes of lower gastrointestinal (GI) bleeding are self-limited and not hemodynamically significant. As with all types of GI bleeding, never neglect it or think it is trivial until a period of vigilant observation tells you whether the bleeding is minor or major, whether it is likely to have ceased or is protracted.

Sources of Bleeding

Probably, many episodes of overt colonic bleeding never have the precise site and cause established. Often the bleeding must be assumed to originate from an already known pathology or maybe simply a guess. Later, when the bleeding episode is over, the diagnostic workup may reveal a previously unknown pathology as the cause or suggest, in retrospect, a lesion that may have been the source. Table 24.1 shows the most common causes (without ranking their relative frequency).

A short comment about the causes mentioned in the table may help you to choose the most likely cause in your next patient with colonic bleeding. *Neoplasms*, whether cancer or benign polyp, rarely bleed massively but often have occult bleeding which can produce significant anemia. A patient with rectal cancer rarely bleeds overtly and if associated with anemia it can at first suggest a massive bleed until rectoscopy is performed. The patient with rectal cancer will give a history of tenesmus and usually there has been episodic minor bleeding with the stools for

Table 24.1. Causes of colorectal bleeding

- Neoplasms
- Inflammatory bowel disease
- Diverticulosis – diverticulitis
- Ischemic colitis
- Vascular malformation – angiodysplasia
- Hemorrhoids
- Postoperative – anastomotic
- Meckel's diverticulum
- Infectious

some time. Bleeding in *inflammatory bowel disease* (IBD) is almost never the first symptom of disease and is rarely massive (chapter 20). The diagnosis will be known in most such patients and the bleeding is associated with an exacerbation, where diarrhea precedes the bleeding by several days. The exception is proctitis which may present with bleeding, again easily identified at rectoscopy. The differential diagnosis of proctitis includes *infections* such as Campylobacter or Amebiasis. The onset is then more sudden with diarrhea and bleeding beginning together just a few days previously.

    Diverticula of the sigmoid colon are assumed to be a common cause of acute major bleeding. By nature it occurs more often in elderly patients, and particularly in those taking non-steroidal anti-inflammatory drugs (NSAID) or anti-coagulants. In middle aged and elderly patients, you must also consider mucosal *angiodysplasia* as a possible explanation for massive and recurrent bleeding. In elderly patients *ischemic colitis* can rarely present with a massive bleeding. *Postoperative* bleeding from colonic anastomoses, polypectomy site, or after anal surgery, should be easily diagnosed. And finally, do not forget that internal hemorrhoids may bleed copiously: you do not want to diagnose an anal source at laparotomy.

Diagnosis

We find it very annoying to consult on bleeding patients where the referral notes simply states: "Patient has melena". Anything can hide behind such a note. It tells us that not a lot of thought was invested in this request. There are two very powerful tools to help you: the patient's history and the rectoscope. First, find out whether the blood is pink-fresh blood, or maroon – almost fresh blood. The later two represent *hemtochezia* (bloody stools) and signify a colonic (common) or small bowel (rare) source. We must not remind you that tarry black stools of *melena* signify an upper gastrointestinal (UGI) source – above the ligament of Treitz (chapter 12). Remember that with massive UGI hemorrhage, and rapid intestinal transit, unaltered fresh blood may appear in the rectum. Insertion of a nasogastric tube with gastric irrigation may quickly direct you to a gastric bleed but remember that bleeding duodenal ulcers may not show blood in the stomach (chapter 12).

Rectoscopy

For all cases of hematochezia the rectoscopy is the first step. It is amazing how often this step is omitted in "modern" practice – how often we see patients immediately referred instead for a "panendoscopy". Use a rigid rectoscope as the flexible instrument will be marred with blood and you will see nothing. Have a good suction device available. It is not unusual that there is simply too much blood to really see anything. If blood can be aspirated and you do get to see the rectum, simple things like a rectal cancer or proctitis should be obvious. Do not decide on a diagnosis of proctitis too lightly because the mucosa may look all red from the fresh blood. The mucosa should be swollen and there should be no visible mucosal blood vessels. The proctitis is often so distal that the margin between inflamed and normal mucosa can be seen. The more red is the blood the closer to the anus is the source. Bleeding from the upper anal canal and lower rectum will reflux at least to the recto-sigmoid junction, so do not be fooled by finding fresh blood at that level. If you have a good view, when there is not too much bleeding, fresh blood may be seen flowing on the wall or dripping from above – in which case bleeding from a more proximal source is likely. Occasionally, in patients with active bleeding you won't be able to see much at rectoscopy. But at least you had the opportunity to exclude an anal source and to personally observe the character and magnitude of the bleeding.

Let us forget at this stage the majority of patients in whom the bleeding stops spontaneously. They will be further investigated with a colonoscopy performed in a well-prepared bowel. Let us concentrate instead on that problematic minority of patients, who bleed massively or continue to bleed. In such patients more aggressive means will be needed to establish and treat the source of the bleeding

The "Sophisticated" Means of Diagnosis

There are two means of diagnosis in this situation: *a technetium-labeled erythrocyte scan* and a *mesenteric angiography*. Which of the two should be chosen roughly depends on the intensity of the bleeding. The more profuse the bleeding – the better it is to start with angiography. Not only will it define the site of the bleeding but also the bleeding vessel may be treated through the angiographic catheter. Both investigations require that the patient is bleedings actively; do not waste the radiologist's time with a non-bleeding patient.

The Operation

Very rarely will the bleeding be so massive that an emergency operation is required to stop the bleeding. *If you have no clue about the pathology the most likely site is angiodysplasia of the right colon.* Make a quick examination of the colon to exclude obvious pathology. Then inspect the small bowel, which may contain blood even if the bleeding comes from the right colon. But it would be unusual for the blood to regurgitate throughout the entire small bowel. If you find blood in the upper small bowel direct your investigation to the upper GI tract. Blood in the right colon, but not small bowel, does not definitely identify the bleeding as being in the right colon because blood will regurgitate long distances. Make your guess based on what you find because now comes the really difficult part. Are you going to take a chance on a right hemicolectomy or can you identify the bleeding spot with certainty? To be sure about the bleeding site you will have to open and clean the colon. It is messy and takes time which is a reason why traditional teaching propose the blind right hemicolectomy. There are instances when the colon is so full with blood that a total or subtotal colectomy is advisable. Temporary clamping of the three main vessels to the colon will reduce the bleeding while you mobilize the colon.

219

Balancing Comment

Not that I disagree with the above contribution by PO Nystrom. It is only that my own experience with, and perception of, lower GI bleeding – slightly differs from his. This is understandable if one realizes that all published data on this topic represent retrospective studies on poorly stratified patents. So this is what I think:

- Let's face it: in nine-tenth of patients with lower GI bleeding the bleeding stops spontaneously. Emergency localizing tests are unnecessary in this group; elective colonoscopy is indicated. Hysterical MD's tend however to over investigate this group – jumping on them with isotope scans and angiograms – all useless when the hemorrhage is not active.
- Each of us operates perhaps once or twice a year on "massive" lower GI bleed (>than 4–6 units bleed over 24 hours – which continues).

Therefore, the collective experience of each hospital is small – not allowing any meaningful prospective studies. All that is published on this subject is therefore retrospective and biased by local dogma and facilities.

- Reports by radiologists that isotope-scans or angiography has that and this accuracy rates are often meaningless, because such reports do not bring up the clinical benefit of such accuracy – e.g. did it change the management and how?
- Essentially most "massive" lower GI bleedings in elderly patients are either from colonic diverticula (in the left as well as the right colon) and angiodysplasia (on the right side). True, angiodysplasia lesions are common but we do not know how often they bleed. It is my impression that colonoscopists often over-diagnose these lesions as the source after the hemorrhage has ceased, whereas the true source of bleeding was elsewhere (e.g. diverticular).

Based on the above considerations this is how I would approach a LGI bleed:

- Start with supportive care. Exclude upper GI bleeding. There is no need for a routine upper GI endoscopy, as fresh blood per rectum in a stable patient means that the source is not in the upper GI tract. Do a rectoscopy to rule out an anorectal source.
- When the patient requires the second and third unit of blood – I am starting to get a little excited. Angiography at this stage is indicated – if it localizes the source of bleeding in the left or right colon – I am happy. If it fails – not a big deal. Isotope scan requires time and is clinically almost useless in actively bleeding patients. Blood migrates within the lumen of the colon and so the extravasated isotope.
- When the patient is on his 5th or sixth unit and blood is still dripping from his rectum – it is time to take him to the operating room. If angiography has localized the source in either the left or right

colon I do a segmental colectomy – either right or left hemicolectomy. If angiography is not available or non-localizing I do subtotal
colectomy. "Blind" segmental colectomy may produce a re-bleeder
who won't tolerate a major re-operation. I do not think that
subtotal colectomy should have a higher mortality than hemicolectomy – see the excellent results of subtotal colectomy in patients
with left colonic obstruction (chapter 21).

- A few authors have described intra-operative colonoscopy after an
  'on table' colonic lavage. Theoretically it appears attractive but
  practically it is messy and time consuming. If the hemorrhage has
  stopped it won't show us much: try and see what is an angiodysplasia and what is just some old clotted blood.

- There is no doubt that in practice we are over-investigating those
  patients and often waiting too long prior to operation. The bleeding
  either stops or continues; when it continues you must operate – on
  a well-resuscitated patient who has not been allowed to deteriorate
  in a medical ward. A fast subtotal colectomy is a safe, definitive,
  and life saving procedure.

Whether I am right or wrong depends on which papers you read, on
what you believe, your local facilities and your own philosophy. I hope
you'll adopt mine.

> **Beware: in lower gastrointestinal bleeding,**
> **removing the wrong side of the colon is embarrassing.**
> **Removing any segment of the colon**
> **while the bleeding source is in the colorectum**
> **is shameful.**

25 Gynecological Emergencies

*Have you ever seen a gynecologist who is convinced
that the "acute abdomen" is gynecological in origin,
and not due to acute appendicitis?*

As a practicing general surgeon you are unlikely to deliver a baby but
likely to face a gynecological problem that you should know how to han-
dle. Acute abdominal pain is very common in women during their reproductive age. Such pain commonly is "gynecological" in origin but it may
as likely be "surgical". Your gynecological colleagues are generally "nice"
but typically posses a vision limited by the boundaries of the bony pelvis.
Consequently, they are often reluctant to diagnose any acute condition
as "gynecological" unless you have ruled-out acute appendicitis.
Occasionally you operate for what you think is acute appendicitis and
the findings are "gynecological". You should know how to deal with it.
Another situation, which provides you with the pleasure of interacting
with gynecologists-obstetricians, is the pregnant patient. As you know –
pregnancy by itself may be the cause of abdominal pain while at the
same time it may modify the presentation of common surgical disorders,
making diagnosis difficult. It may also pose considerable challenges in
the injured patient.

Acute Abdominal Pain in the Fertile Woman

Assessment & Approach

We do not have to remind you to take a history concerning *menstruation,
sexual activity* and *contraception*. Pregnancy, be it uterine or *ectopic*,
should be always ruled out; this is done in most hospitals with a rapid
pregnancy test. History of pain, which occurs during the first days of the

224 menstrual period, hints to underlying *endometriosis* or *endometrioma* ("chocolate cyst"). Acute pain, which develops at the mid-menstrual cycle (*mittelschmerz*), points to a rupture of the Graafian follicle at ovulation. Pain referred to the shoulder suggests the possibility of *free intra-peritoneal blood* – irritating the diaphragm; the source of the blood may be a *ruptured ovarian cyst or an ectopic pregnancy*.

There is also no need to talk with you about physical examination. You surely know that the conditions to be discussed below can produce signs of peritoneal irritation, often indistinguishable from that of acute appendicitis. *The site of pain and local findings on examination* are helpful in narrowing the differential diagnosis: when bilateral – consider pelvic inflammatory disease (*PID*), when on the right think about acute appendicitis, when on the left, in an older lady, consider acute diverticulitis (chapter 2).

By now your gynecological friend has performed a bimanual vaginal examination. You can do it also yourself – palpating for masses or fullness at the cul-de-sac and looking for "*excitation tenderness* – when moving the cervix produces a lot of pain (PID, ectopic pregnancy). Your friend hopefully is also armed with a trans-vaginal ultrasound, allowing him to visualize free fluid, the uterus and adnexa. When fluid is present at the cul-de-sac, it can be aspirated with a needle through the vagina (*culdocentesis*); *when pus is present think about PID or perforated appendicitis*, while *blood hints to a ruptured cyst or ectopic pregnancy*.

Generally speaking most acute painful gynecological conditions are treated non-operatively. With all the above information at hand, your job now, together with the gynecologist, is to classify the patient into one of the following groups:
- "Benign" abdominal examination; most probably a gynecological condition – *treat conservatively*.
- "Impressive" abdominal examination, no apparent gynecological pathology. This is perhaps the best indication to start with a diagnostic/therapeutic laparoscopy.
- "Not sure". Admit & observe +/- a CT scan. (chapters 2 & 22)

The most common "acute" gynecological problems are complicated ovarian   225
cysts, ectopic pregnancy, and PID. You should know how to diagnose those
conditions, how to treat it conservatively and what to do, if encountered
during laparoscopy or laparotomy – when your old gynecological buddy
is not around or takes hours to arrive.

Ovarian Cysts

"Functional" cysts (follicular or corpum luteum) are common and usually
asymptomatic. Typical features on trans-vaginal ultrasound include:
solitary, no solid components, and size <5 cm. *Acute pain develops when
the cyst ruptures or undergoes torsion.* Rupture with minimal local and
systemic findings should be treated conservatively. If, however, the
rupture results in significant intra-peritoneal hemorrhage and when
another pathology cannot be ruled out – laparoscopy or laparotomy are
indicated. If there is active bleeding from the cyst, obtain local hemostasis
by whichever means. There is no need to aspirate or resect the cyst and
please, do not even think of removing the ovary. *Torsion* is usually associated with more severe pain, abdominal findings and systemic manifestations, calling for a laparoscopy or laparotomy. If viable, the tube and
ovary can be de-torted and conserved; if non-viable – resect.

Ectopic Pregnancy

'Ectopic' means that the fertilized ova got implanted somewhere outside
the usual location (i.e. uterus). The most common site for 'ectopic' are
the tubes but it may occur in the ovary, cervix and abdominal cavity. The
presentation of these patients varies tremendously, the most common
being with an abdominal pain and vaginal bleeding. Many women do
not even know about their pregnancy, ignoring associated symptoms of
pregnancy such as a missed menstruation period. The spectrum of clinical
manifestations is wide, ranging from local lower abdominal pain to

226   diffuse peritonitis with hypovolemic shock. The constellation of clinical picture together with a positive pregnancy test, and empty uterus on ultrasound, confirm the diagnosis.

As a general surgeon you are more likely to be involved with the more dramatic scenario of ruptured tubal (at the isthmus) 'ectopic', which typically occurs as early as the 4th week of gestation. The sudden development of acute peritonitis and hypovolemic shock will force you to rush to the operation room without the gynecologist. Evacuate the gestational sac, control the bleeding sites with suture-ligatures and preserve the ovary. Less dramatic presentations are usually dealt by or with the gynecologist, usually laparoscopically. Note that in most 'ectopics' at operation the bleeding has already stopped; when it is active it may necessitate a simple salpingectomy. When the ovaries are left intact the patient can still undergo in vitro fertilization even after bilateral salpingectomies.

Pelvic Inflammatory Disease (PID)

This is an infective syndrome which involves to a lesser or greater extent, the endometrium, tubes and ovaries. The clinical spectrum of infection is wide, ranging from minimal pain, dyspareunia, fever, and vaginal discharge, associated with mild endometritis/salphigitis, to severe peritonitis and septic shock due to ruptured tubo-ovarian abscess. Likewise, physical findings depend on the disease process and vary from localized abdominal tenderness to generalized tenderness and rebound. Note that the pain and tenderness are commonly *bilateral*. Pelvic examination reveals purulent discharge with cervical motion tenderness. Ovarian or pelvic abscess may be palpated or seen on ultrasound or CT. The majority of "mild cases" should be treated with antibiotics. Outpatient treatment is appropriate for patients who can tolerate oral diet. Patients with severe abdominal and systemic manifestation should be admitted for intravenous antibiotic therapy. Antibiotic treatment is "empiric", targeting the

common causative organisms which are, in isolation or combination,   227
C.*trachomatis, N. gonorrhea, E. coli, and H. influenza*.. Many oral and I.V. agents are available for you to choose from.

Patients who do not respond to the above regimen or in whom the diagnosis is uncertain are subjected to laparoscopy. This should be left to the gynecologist. The typical case you will be involved with is the ruptured tubo-ovarian abscess, causing severe pelvic or diffuse peritonitis. During laparotomy or laparoscopy you'll find pus; how to deal with peritonitis you read in chapter 10. The abscess should be drained, whether to remove the uterus and ovaries depends on the age of the patient, the operative findings and your gynecologist.

When talking about PID, "formal" textbooks usually would mention *the Curtis-Fitz-Hugh syndrome* or "perihepatitis" as a late sequel – ascending from the pelvis. Although originally associated with *gonococcal* infection, nearly all present-day cases are associated with *C. trachomatis* infection. It may produce non-specific abdominal complains and has been reported to mimic acute cholecystitis, but in our experience hitherto it has never represented a specific entity warranting operative measures. We have seen it however as an incidental finding of peri-hepatic "piano-string" adhesions at laparoscopy or laparotomy for other conditions.

Acute Abdominal Pain in the Pregnant Women

General Considerations

Abdominal emergencies in pregnant women pose a great challenge to us general surgeons because of the following reasons:

- The ascending uterus gradually distorts the normal abdominal anatomy, displacing organs and thus changing the "typical" clinical scenario.

- Physiologically, the pregnant woman is different: nausea and vomiting are not uncommon during the first trimester, thereafter, tachycardia, mild elevation of temperature and leukocytosis are considered "normal".
- To a certain degree, abdominal "pains and aches" are common during pregnancy.
- When dealing with a sick pregnant women you automatically have two patients – the life and well being of the fetus has also to be considered.

Generally speaking acute abdominal conditions during pregnancy are either:
- *Specific to pregnancy.*
- *Concidentally developing during pregnancy.*

Abdominal Emergencies Specific to Pregnancy

Abdominal emergencies specific to pregnancy are either:
- *"Obstetric"* – such as ectopic pregnancy (see above), abortion and septic abortion (a "septic" uterus may present with an impressive 'acute abdomen'), "red degeneration" of a fibroid, abruptio placenta, rupture of uterus, and pre-eclampsia. These conditions won't be further discussed. Hey, we did not promise you a manual of obstetrics.
- *"General"*-such as acute pyelonephritis, which is more common in pregnant women or rupture of visceral aneurysm (i.e. splenic) which is rare but "typically" occurring during pregnancy. Another condition, which may be associated with pregnancy, is a *spontaneous hematoma of the rectus abdominis muscle.* (This condition may also develop in non-pregnant women – and even men for that matter – in particular in anti-coagulated patients). The hematoma originates from a ruptured branch of the inferior epigastric artery

and develops deep to the muscle. On examination a tender   229
abdominal-wall mass is often felt; it won't disappear when the
patient tenses his or her abdominal wall (Fothergill's sign).
Ultrasound or a CT can confirm the diagnosis. Treatment is
conservative.

Abdominal Emergencies Concidentally Developing During Pregnancy

Any abdominal emergency may occur during pregnancy. Here are a few
basic considerations:

- *Think "in trimesters"*: during the *first trimester* the fetus is most
  susceptible to the potential damaging effects of drugs and X-rays.
  Abdominal operations in this stage may precipitate an abortion.
  Operations during the *third trimester* are more likely to induce a
  pre-mature labor, posing additional risk to the mother and fetus.
  Thus, surgery is *best tolerable during the second trimester* – if you
  have the luxury of choice.
- *The well being of the mother overrides that of the fetus.* If maternal
  and fetal distress is present simultaneously on presentation, all
  therapeutic efforts should be towards the mother. A C-section is
  considered only if the fetus is more than 24 weeks old and in
  persistent distress in spite of maximal therapy to the mother.
- *Pregnant women suffer from a chronic abdominal compartment
  syndrome (chapter 28).* The abdominal emergency (e.g. perforated
  appendicitis or intestinal obstruction) will further increase the
  intra-abdominal pressure, reducing venous return and cardiac output. Place such patients in *a left lateral decubitus position* in order
  to shift the gravid uterus away from the compressed inferior vena
  cava.

230   You should be aware of:

- *Acute appendicitis.* You are commonly called to "exclude acute appendicitis" in a pregnant women. Address the problem as discussed in chapter 22, but be aware that as the pregnancy advances, the cecum, with the attached appendix, is displaced proximally and laterally – towards where the gallbladder is. In addition, the appendix shifts progressively beyond the protective, "walling-off" reach of the omentum – making free perforation more likely. An ultrasound may help in excluding acute cholecystitis. Diagnostic laparoscopy and/or laparoscopic appendectomy during pregnancy were reported safe to the mother and fetus but still remain somehow controversial. If you choose to operate, tilt the table to left and places a muscle splitting incision *directly over the point of maximal tenderness* – wherever it is.

- *Acute cholecystitis.* This is easily recognized clinically and ultrasonographically (chapter 15) also during pregnancy. During the first trimester try conservative management, delaying the operation to the second trimester. If occurring during the third trimester try to postpone the operation, if possible, until after the delivery. Laparoscopic cholecystectomy appears safe during pregnancy. This is perhaps the place to mention the *HELLP Syndrome* (Hemolysis, Elevated Liver enzymes, and Low Platelet count). It is a relatively rare syndrome, which may develop in a pre-eclamptic, pre-term, patient and be confused with acute biliary disease (even a "mild" HELLP may stretch the liver capsule producing severe RUQ pain). Liver hemorrhage and hematoma and even liver rupture are serious complications of the HELLP syndrome and represent a surgical emergency: the child should be promptly delivered and the liver managed based on "trauma principles" – in the unstable, coagulopathic patient the liver should be packed (chapter 27). Think about HELLP – a misguided cholecystectomy may kill the mother and her offspring.

- *Intestinal obstruction: sigmoid* or *cecal volvulus* is more common   231
  during late pregnancy. The displacement of abdominal structures
  during pregnancy may also "shift" "stable" adhesions, producing
  small bowel obstruction or volvulus. Pregnancy tends to "cloud"
  presenting features and impedes early diagnosis. Notice that a few
  plain abdominal X- rays, with or without Gastrografin (chapters 3,
  7 & 21), are entirely safe even in early pregnancy; so if you suspect
  a large or small bowel obstruction – do not hesitate. Remember
  that intestinal strangulation threatens the life of the mother and
  her prospective child.

Trauma in Pregnancy

The management of abdominal trauma in pregnancy is identical to the
management in the non-pregnant woman (chapters 26 & 27), except that
in pregnancy there is concern for two patients: the mother and the fetus.
Therefore, assessment of the fetal status by either by Doppler or by
continuous cardiotocodynamometry is mandatory when the clinical
circumstances permit. The major clinical concerns in the injured pregnant
female are uterine rupture and abruptio placentae. The former condition
is suggested by abdominal tenderness and signs of peritoneal irritation,
sometimes in conjunction with palpable fetal parts or inability to palpate
the fundus. The latter is suggested by vaginal bleeding and uterine con-
tractions. When the fetus is in jeopardy, a rapid caesarian section is
usually in the best interests of both the mother and fetus.

The "Post-partum" Period

Abdominal emergencies are notoriously difficult to diagnose during the
early post-partum or post C-section period. Abdominal pain and
gastrointestinal symptoms are commonly attributed to "after pain", and
fever or systemic malaise to "residual endometritis". In addition, at this

232   phase the abdominal wall is maximally stretched out and redundant, not
able to elicit guarding and other peritoneal signs. Things "move around"
the abdomen during delivery and a loop of bowel may be twisted or
caught. We have treated perforated acute appendicitis, perforated peptic
ulcer and acute cholecystitis during the early post partum days.
Diagnosis is usually delayed and so is the treatment. Be aware!

26 Penetrating Abdominal Trauma

It is absolutely necessary for a surgeon to search the wounds himself,
which were not drest by him at first,
in order to discover their nature and know their extent
(A.Belloste)

Clinical is better and cheaper than high tech

To Operate or Not To Operate?

The key decision you will be faced with is whether an exploratory
laparotomy is required. The decision to operate usually means that you
will proceed to the operating room immediately, while the decision *not*
to operate is subject to frequent reassessment in the next 24 (rarely 48)
hours. You decide to operate because you presume that there is significant
intra-abdominal injury to repair, but you may be wrong. *A laparotomy is
termed "negative" if no injuries were present and "non-therapeutic" if the
injuries would have healed without surgical intervention*; for example,
hemoperitoneum from a self-limited minor hepatic tear. Since both
negative and non-therapeutic laparotomies are not entirely harmless, it
should be your aim not to operate unnecessarily. Unfortunately, this is
often easier said than done.

After penetrating abdominal trauma, two possible clinical pictures
can be found, in isolation or in combination: *hypovolemic shock and/or
peritonitis.* The former is the result of intra-abdominal bleeding caused
by the injury of a solid organ (liver, spleen, kidney) or of a sizeable
blood vessel; the latter is the result of an injury to a hollow viscus (gut,
urinary bladder, biliary system) with subsequent soiling of the peritoneal
cavity.

There are two main mechanisms of penetrating abdominal trauma:
stab wounds and gunshot injuries. Traditionally, the two decision-making

234   algorithms have differed; more recently, there has been a tendency to apply the same approach in both types of injury.

Stab Wounds

The diagnosis of a stabbed abdomen is straightforward in the majority of patients: there is a visible wound on the abdominal wall and the patient or witnesses usually confirm the circumstances of the assault. Occasionally, you will see evisceration of abdominal content (usually omentum or small bowel) through the stab wound, and rarely the patient will be brought to the ER with the wounding agent still in place.

The indications for laparotomy in patients with abdominal stab wounds are pretty straightforward. If the patient shows signs of either *hemodynamic instability* (in the absence of an associated injury that can account for shock) or *peritonitis*, the indication for laparotomy is obvious. If there is evisceration of abdominal content or the wounding agent is protruding, the decision is easy too. It is the *asymptomatic* patient with an abdominal stab wound that the decision to operate is more problematic. Of these asymptomatic patients, about one third do not even have peritoneal penetration, and another third do not have significant abdominal injury. Thus operating on all patients with an abdominal stab wound would not be a good idea.

Your decision to operate, taken on either of these two findings, is a *clinical decision*. It does not require further confirmation by an abdominal roentgenogram, diagnostic peritoneal lavage, contrast studies, ultrasound or CT scans, or worst of all, diagnostic laparoscopy; nor, indeed, can it be replaced by any of these tests. *Clinical evaluation is the most reliable method of diagnosing significant penetrating intra-abdominal injuries*; the resort to expensive or time-consuming investigations is mostly unnecessary for either diagnostic or medico-legal purposes.

The only useful investigations in this setting are intravenous
pyelography and retrograde cystography in the presence of hematuria;
the aim here is not so much to determine the necessity for an operation,
but rather the type and level of injury to the urinary tract (and, most
importantly, the presence of two functioning kidneys).

235

Selective Conservatism

The Absence of Shock or Peritonitis Justifies
a Non-operative Approach, at Least Initially

The concept of observation implies an attentive and sustained commitment
to this patient:

- An intravenous access is secured.
- A Foley catheter is inserted to monitor the urine output, and more
  importantly to avoid a spurious diagnosis of peritonitis caused by
  a distended bladder (try to press on your own lower abdomen
  after the ingestion of a couple of pints of beer).
- The vital signs are charted initially half-hourly, then hourly, to
  detect early shock.
- The abdomen is frequently re-evaluated at intervals of 1–3 hours,
  preferably by the same surgeon. Note: the stab wound and its
  surroundings are usually tender. It is useful to mark with a pen the
  tender zone around the laceration to monitor for subsequent
  spread of the tenderness beyond the marked area. Even if you feel
  that the patient may object to being treated as a drawing table, the
  underlying principle is to look for evidence of tenderness *away
  from the stab wound*.
- Nasogastric decompression, analgesics or antibiotics are not
  required.

236   The non-operative option is then considered to have been applied successfully when no shock or peritonitis has been uncovered within the 24–36 hours from the time of assault. Keep an open mind at all times; do not try to prove a point by persevering with non-operative management in the face of even subtle deterioration. Having to operate after an initial period of unsuccessful observation is not a sign of personal failure but of good clinical skills. Much has been written on the morbidity of negative laparotomies. The complications of a negative trauma laparotomy, especially in the context of penetrating trauma where associated extra-abdominal injuries are infrequent, have been grossly exaggerated. A negative laparotomy for penetrating trauma is nothing to be ashamed of, and when in doubt it is safest for the patient to err on the side of caution.

Note: people who perform unnecessary investigations on patients with stab wounds to the abdomen do it because they lack clinical skills and experience. In our hands, and that of others, the clinical approach has proven reliable and safe. Do you want to be known as a seasoned clinician? Practice it.

Gunshot Wounds

There is a much greater likelihood of significant intra-abdominal injuries in gunshot than in stab wounds. Traditional wisdom has held that a gunshot wound mandates an exploratory laparotomy, irrespective of the patient's clinical condition. There has been recently a growing body of opinion that these injuries, when asymptomatic, can be managed along the same lines as stab wounds. It is probably a good idea to obtain an abdominal X-ray on these patients to see the trajectory of the bullet. A trajectory that crosses the abdominal midline may indicate a silent vertebral or even major vascular injury. A missing bullet should prompt a search for a hidden exit wound or a bullet embolism. Consequently the occasionol clinically – "innocent" abdomen in a hemodynamically stable patient can be observed, like in the stab scenario.

Difficult Scenarios

Penetrating injuries to the *lower chest*, the *buttocks* or the *perineum* pose the problem of possible and unsuspected penetration of the abdominal cavity. An isolated diaphragmatic laceration is usually clinically silent initially but has to be nevertheless diagnosed if secondary complications (diaphragmatic hernia) are to be avoided; diagnostic peritoneal lavage, thoracoscopy or laparoscopy may be useful adjuncts in low thoracic injuries for the assessment of diaphragmatic integrity. In fact, this is the only indication we know for laparoscopy in abdominal injury! Note however that the natural history of post-traumatic diaphragmatic defects is unknown; it may be that if "missed" – most will remain silent forever. More on laparoscopy in trauma see chapter 41.

Similarly, the breach of the pelvic floor as a result of a gluteal or perineal injury and intra-abdominal penetration may give rise to delayed clinical presentation and morbidity: diagnostic peritoneal lavage may detect peritoneal penetration at an early stage and help in decision-making.

Stab wounds of the *loins* have the potential for injury to the posterior colonic wall, which may result in massive retroperitoneal infection if left undetected. Peritoneal signs are present only at a late stage (sometimes too late). The use of a contrast enema coupled with CT scanning may be helpful; alternatively, mandatory exploration can be advocated at the price of a high proportion of negative laparotomies.

To review exploration of the abdomen consult chapter 9.

To recapitulate: the two cardinal principles in exploration for penetrating trauma are:

- The number of holes in the GI tract must be paired, because an unpaired number raises the probability of a missed injury.
  Although it is possible to have a "tangential" penetration or to have the missile lodge inside the bowel, this is less common then a missed injury.
- The trajectory of the wounding missile (i.e. sequence of injured organs) should "make sense". You must be able to construct a logical mental picture of the bullet trajectory, because if the trajectory is non-continuous of non-linear, you must suspect a missed injury.

About injuries to *specific organs* look at chapter 27.

**It is highly desirable that anyone engaged
in war surgery should keep his idea fluid
and so be ready to abandon methods
which prove unsatisfactory in favor of others which,
at first, may appear revolutionary
and even not free from inherent danger
(H.H Sampson, 1940)**

27 Blunt Abdominal Trauma

It is more difficult to decide
when not to operate
than when to operate
and what operation to perform

The Need to Supplement
the Clinical Evaluation

Blunt abdominal trauma is different from penetrating trauma on several counts:

- Penetrating trauma is identified by the presence of an abdominal wound; blunt abdominal trauma is merely suspected or inferred.
- While penetrating trauma is usually unicavitary (i.e. absent extra-abdominal injuries), blunt trauma is usually part of a multi-cavity injury complex. The presence of other injuries may mask abdominal symptoms or signs: for example, the pain produced by a flail thoracic segment or by long bone fractures is a strong confounding factor in distorting the patient's perception of abdominal pain or tenderness, and diverting the clinician's attention from the abdomen.
- A decreased level of consciousness (due to a head injury or alcohol) is often present in blunt polytrauma, rendering communication with the patient impossible and clinical abdominal evaluation unreliable.
- Blunt trauma causes intra-abdominal bleeding and shock much more frequently than peritonitis from a hollow visceral injury. Hemorrhagic shock in this context is often ascribed, quite plausibly, to extra-abdominal sources of bleeding; these are often present: long bone or pelvic fractures, a hemothorax or peripheral vascular injuries.

240   For all these reasons, the reliance on clinical pictures of shock or peritonitis cannot constitute the sole foundation for deciding on a laparotomy
in blunt trauma. Additional diagnostic modalities are indispensable.
Three such tools play a crucial role in the decision to operate or not to
operate: diagnostic peritoneal lavage (DPL), CT scan and ultrasound
(US). Which of the three you use as the chief diagnostic tool depends of
course on your local circumstances and facilities.

Diagnostic Peritoneal Lavage (DPL)

DPL has been the gold standard in evaluating blunt abdominal trauma.
It aims at detecting the presence of free blood in the peritoneal cavity.
Gross blood aspirated from the intraperitoneal catheter or a red cell
count of over 100,000/mm^3 constitute a positive lavage. The threshold
of 10,000/mm^3 is a very low one and it corresponds to the presence of
only a few milliliters of free intraperitoneal blood. A clear return (a
negative lavage) excludes the presence of intra-peritoneal injury. You
should never blame yourself for the performance of a DPL that turns out
to be negative: this is a valuable piece of information in a polytrauma
patient.

A positive lavage is extremely reliable in uncovering the presence
of intraperitoneal hemorrhage. At laparotomy in patients with a positive
lavage an intra-peritoneal blood is always found. The weakness of the
DPL lies however in it being *hypersensitive*: many sources of bleeding are
self-limiting and do not require surgical control (e.g. a small omental
tear or even more substantial injuries of the liver or spleen). A laparotomy
in these patients is termed *"non-therapeutic"*. Compared with the negative
laparotomy for penetrating trauma it tends to cause a greater morbidity,
as it is performed usually in the settings of multiple extra-abdominal
injuries.

The Major Indications for DPL

- The physical examination of the patient is unreliable, usually due to an altered level of consciousness.
- The patient cannot be frequently reassessed because he or she requires an operative procedure on another anatomical region (e.g. craniotomy or bone-fixation) and will thus be lost to follow up for many hours.

Abdominal Computerized Tomography (CT)

CT scan of the abdomen provides excellent visual information on both peritoneal and retroperitoneal structures, and is the key imaging modality in stable patients with blunt abdominal trauma. A CT scan takes at least forty minutes from the minute you decide to have it done until you see the pictures on the monitor. Therefore, it is contra-indicated in unstable patients. By localizing the injury to one or other solid intra-abdominal organ, the abdominal CT scan enables the better-informed surgeon to opt for non-operative management, provided the patient remains or is easily kept hemodynamically stable. It must be noted that CT scan is notoriously deficient in imaging appropriately hollow visceral injuries, which are, however, rare in blunt trauma.

Abdominal Ultrasound (US)

US is emerging as a serious contender to DPL in the evaluation of blunt abdominal trauma. Performed in the trauma resuscitation area by a member of the trauma team, it aims at rapid diagnosis of free intra-peritoneal fluid (usually blood) rather than at the identification of specific organ injury (this highly questionable endeavor should be left to radiologists whose opinions should be often politely disregarded).

242   Philosophy of Non-operative Approach in Blunt Trauma

For the hemodynamically stable patient with a non-tender abdomen and CT evidence of trauma to the spleen or liver, non-operative management is becoming an increasingly popular option. However, the prudent surgeon must realize that there is a fundamental difference between these two organs.

Liver

For the hemodynamically stable patient with a significant liver injury diagnosed by CT scan, non-operative management is a very attractive option because it can save the patient a surgical procedure that may easily "turn sour". Exploration and adequate mobilization of the injured liver may lead to a situation where bleeding will be controlled with difficulty, often with peri-hepatic packing which, while life-saving, is associated with greatly increased morbidity. Regardless of the anatomical configuration of the injury, if:

- the patient is hemodynamically stable
- the abdomen is non-tender
- there is only a very small amount of free blood in the peritoneal cavity

then non-operative management is reasonably safe – provided that the patient can be closely watched in a monitored environment and that preparations have been made for rapid transfer to the operating room should the need arise. If the patient complains of sudden abdominal pain or if there is hepatic tenderness or increase in the size of the palpable liver, then hemostasis is required. Selective angiographic embolization of branches of the hepatic arteries is an important adjunct to non-operative management, but is not applicable in the collapsing patient who requires an immediate laparotomy.

Spleen

Non-operative management of splenic injuries is also a valid option, but its benefits are less clear-cut then with the liver. Splenectomy is a low-morbidity procedure when performed in a timely fashion, and the long term threat of overwhelming post-splenectomy infection pertains mainly to the pediatric age group. For adults undergoing splenectomy for trauma the risk of overwhelming infection is negligible. Thus, while non-operative management of the injured spleen is a valid alternative, the prudent surgeon should have no hesitation in proceeding with laparotomy and either splenic repair or splenectomy with the first sign of possible hemo-dynamic deterioration or a questionable finding on physical examination of the abdomen. The risks of blood transfusions may be higher than that of a splenectomy!

Remember: because the morbidity of an unnecessary laparotomy in blunt trauma is not negligible, the low threshold for intervention that is indicated in penetrating abdominal trauma cannot be applied unthinkingly in this context. The decision to proceed with a laparotomy in a blunt polytrauma patient rests on an intelligent use of diagnostic modalities and on the knowledge of their pitfalls. Most patients with blunt abdominal injury can, and should, be managed non-operatively.

Management of Individual Organ Injuries

You decided to perform a laparotomy. The incision and finding what's wrong are described in chapters 8 and 9, respectively. Herein, we'll run with you over the essentials in the management of specific abdominal injuries. In general doing "less" in blunt trauma may be "better" – the less blood you loose the better is the outlook for the patient. *Do not forget that your operation and its magnitude add "inflammation" to the SIRS already caused by the polytrauma* (chapter 38).

244   There has been a trend, especially in blunt trauma, to treat certain injuries non-operatively; the indications for such conservative management are discussed above. This section describes, in brief, the intra-operative treatment options for each injured organ, whether intra- or retro-peritoneal.

Diaphragm

A through and through diaphragmatic laceration requires closure with interrupted, heavy, sutures. Lacerations with substantial tissue loss are rare and need repair with a synthetic mesh-patch.

Liver

Bleeding from small, superficial capsular tears can be controlled by diathermy or individual vessel ligation. More severe bleeding constitute a surgical challenge requiring a stepwise approach. Appropriate exposure is the first step, which consists of improving exposure by dividing the falciform ligament and sometimes extending the initial midline abdominal incision into a right subcostal incision or even to the chest by either right thoracotomy or median sternotomy. After initial assessment, bimanual compression of the hepatic parenchyma will control the bleeding temporarily, allowing the anesthetist to catch up will the blood loss. The *Pringle maneuver* (occlusion of the undissected triad of portal vein, hepatic artery and common bile duct) is an essential adjunct; it is safe for a period in excess of 60 minutes. This is followed by the mobilization of the liver by division of its ligamentous attachments. Deep parenchymal bleeding is then controlled by finger fracture technique, individual vessel ligation or clipping, and conservative resectional debridement. Residual parenchymal dead space can be plugged with viable omentum. Occasionally, bleeding cannot be controlled because it is compounded by a coagulopathy; it is in these situations that damage control by packing

may be indicated. Retrohepatic caval injuries are characterized by
exanguinating hemorrhage despite an adequate Pringle maneuver ;
probably there are more techniques described for immediate hemostasis
than there are survivors; it is perhaps best to resort to damage control
with packing and come back to fight another day. Injuries to the porta
hepatis require a wide *Kocher maneuver* for exposure. The injured portal
vein should be ideally repaired or, as a last resort, ligated. Hepatic artery
ligation is better tolerated than portal vein ligation. Suture repair or
Roux-en-Y biliary enteric anastomoses are the treatment options for an
injured common bile duct; the latter can be performed either at the
initial operation or at the reconstruction phase of a damage control
strategy. Unilateral lobar bile duct injuries should be managed by ligation.

Spleen

The treatment at laparotomy of a significant splenic injury in the adult is
splenectomy. The risk for post-splenectomy sepsis exists but it is small
and can be further minimized by adequate prophylaxis and vigilance; it
is nevertheless often overemphasized to justify what we regard as potentially harmful acrobatic surgical maneuvers of splenic conservation.

Kidney and Ureter

The intra-operative discovery of a perinephric hematoma is usually in-
dicative of renal injury, but a large proportion of these are self-limiting.
Kidney exploration is indicated in the presence of an expanding or pulsatile hematoma, or when a hilar injury is suspected. Moderate severity
injuries can be controlled usually by cortical renorrhaphy and drainage;
occasionally, a polar nephrectomy may be indicated. A shattered kidney
or a vascular hilar injury require nephrectomy. Lacerations of the renal
pelvis are treated with fine absorbable sutures. An injured ureter should
be carefully exposed, avoiding ischemic damage by over-enthusiastic

246   skeletonization. Primary repair over a double-j stent with absorbable
material is the rule. Either very proximal or very distal ureteric injuries
require expert urologic opinion.

Pancreas

The anterior aspect of the pancreas is exposed through the lesser sac by
division of the gastrocolic omentum; the posterior aspect of the head is
exposed by a *Kocher maneuver,* while access to the posterior aspect of
the tail is achieved by splenic mobilization. The state of the main pancreatic
duct is a crucial determinant of the operative strategy to the injured
pancreas. Intraoperative pancreatography (through a duodenotomy and
cannulation of the ampulla of Vater) may be helpful in assessing the duct
and is more easily performed than intraoperative endoscopic pancreatography, but in practice, it is very rarely performed. If the main duct
appears intact (superficial parenchymal wounds) most pancreatic injuries
require drainage alone. When deeper parenchymal wounds are observed
in the body or tail, indicating the possibility of a distal ductal transection,
a distal pancreatectomy (usually with splenectomy) is indicated. For
deeper injuries of the head a wide drainage is indicated: the management
of the inevitable pancreatic fistula is simpler than that of a leaking
enteric fistula in the aftermath of a fancy immediate reconstruction with
Roux-en-Y pancreaticojejunostomy. The Whipple procedure is reserved
for massive injuries of the pancreatic head, with common bile duct and
duodenal disruptions; the procedure is attended by a high mortality and
should be "staged" – with the reconstruction performed only after the
patient has been stabilized.

Stomach

Most injuries are caused by penetrating trauma and are treated by simple
suture repair. The posterior gastric wall should always be checked by

opening the lesser sac. Blunt injuries are rare and gastric resection   247
exceptionally required.

Duodenum

Intramural duodenal hematomas without full-thickness injury do not
require evacuation; nasogastric suction, fluid replacement and nutrition
(intravenous or via jejunostomy) need to be instituted for up to 3–4 weeks.
Clean-cut, small lacerations can be safely repaired primarily. Extensive
lacerations, the presence of significant tissue contusion (usually inflicted
by blunt trauma), involvement of the common bile duct, or high velocity
gunshot injuries should be treated by duodenal repair and pyloric
exclusion. This procedure consists of closure of the pylorus through a
gastrotomy and re-establishment of gastrointestinal continuity by a gas-
trojejunostomy; the addition of a truncal vagotomy is not necessary.
A feeding jejunostomy is a useful adjunct, in the absence of contraindications, for the provision of enteral nutrition. The Whipple operation is
reserved for massive combined pancreaticoduodenal disruptions; in an
unstable patient you should stage it-resect first and return another day
for reconstruction.

Small Bowel

Most lacerations can be treated by simple suture repair; occasionally a
segmental resection with end-to-end anastomosis is required for the
treatment of multiple lacerations in close proximity. Neglected,
long-standing small bowel lacerations with severe peritonitis of more
than 18–24 hours duration require the fashioning of small bowel stomas
rather than repair.

248   *Colon*

Right or left-sided lacerations colonic lacerations can be safely treated
by suture repair or resection with primary anastomosis (by necessity, in
an unprepared colon). Long-standing peritonitis mandates the performance of a colostomy. The modern trend has been to avoid a colostomy
even with significant fecal contamination, in the shocked patient or in
the presence of associated multiple intra-abdominal injuries. We believe,
however, that the drawbacks of a colostomy should always be weighed
against the risk of a fecal fistula (sometimes with disastrous consequences)
and the determined avoidance of a colostomy at any price does turn out
to be sometimes a very costly act of surgical bravado.

Rectum

In the absence of gross fecal contamination, minor lacerations can be
repaired by simple suture repair. In all other cases, a proximal diverting
colostomy must be added; a loop sigmoid colostomy is usually adequate.
Wash-out of the distal rectal stump and pre-sacral drainage seem
unnecessary except in extensive injuries with wide dissection and soiling
of the peri-rectal spaces.

Bladder

An intraperitoneal rupture requires repair with absorbable sutures
and catheter drainage; in an extraperitoneal rupture, catheter drainage
alone is sufficient. In both cases, the bladder drainage provided by
a urethral Foley catheter is adequate, rendering suprapubic drainage
unnecessary.

Intra-abdominal Vascular Injuries   249

The most important step in the management of *aortic* injuries is exposure
in order to achieve proximal and distal control (see also chapter 9). The
posterior parietal peritoneum must be incised lateral to the left colon,
allowing the reflection of the colon to the right and the small bowel
medially. If needed, other organs can also be reflected medially: left
kidney, spleen and pancreas, stomach. The suprarenal aorta can be
approached through the gastrocolic omentum, via the lesser sac, with
retraction of the stomach and esophagus to the left. For high injuries,
a left thoracotomy may be required. Aortic injuries require repair with a
3–0 or 4–0 polypropylene monofilament.

The exposure to the *infrahepatic vena cava* is achieved by incision
of the peritoneum lateral to the right colon and medial reflection of the
right colon, duodenum, right kidney and small bowel (see also chapter 9).
The bleeding site must be occluded by direct finger pressure, the use
of sponge-sticks or vascular clamps; no attempt should be made to encircle completely the vessel. Venorrhaphy can be achieved with a 4–0 or
5–0 monofilament vascular suture; also check for the presence of a
posterior laceration that can be repaired by gently rotating the vena cava
or from inside the vessel. In massive disruptions, a synthetic graft may be
used, but more commonly the infrarenal vena cava is ligated.

Injured *common or external iliac arteries* should be repaired; if a
graft is necessary, synthetic material may be used even in the presence of
peritoneal soiling. When the later is however heavy – the artery should
be ligated and circulation restored with a fem-fem extra-anatomic bypass.
The *internal iliac artery* may be ligated with impunity. The exposure of
the *iliac veins* is notoriously difficult and may require the division of the
ipsilateral internal iliac artery or even a temporary division of a common
iliac artery. Iliac veins may be ligated with little morbidity provided
compression stockings and limb elevation is used postoperatively.

The *celiac artery*, the retro-pancreatic portion of the superior mesenteric artery and the inferior mesenteric artery may be ligated; the infra-pancreatic superior mesenteric artery should be repaired. The superior mesenteric vein should be repaired if possible, but ligation causes bowel infarction in a small percentage of cases only. The inferior mesenteric artery may be ligated with impunity.

Retroperitoneal Hematoma

The main issue is whether to explore or observe such a hematoma discovered in the course of a trauma laparotomy. *As a general rule, in penetrating trauma, all retroperitoneal hematomas should be explored, irrespective of their location or size.* In blunt trauma, a more selective policy can be applied, depending mainly on the location of the hematoma. A *central abdominal location (Zone I)* (including the main abdominal vessels and the duodeno-pancreatic complex) always warrants exploration. *Lateral hematomas (Zone II)* (including kidney and retroperitoneal portion of the colon) can be left alone, unless they are very large in size, pulsating or expanding. *Blunt traumatic pelvic hematomas (Zone III)* should not be explored (see Table 27.1).

Table 27.1. Approach to traumatic retroperitoneal hematoma

Type-Hematoma	Penetrating injury	Blunt injury
Central (Zone I)	Explore	Explore
Lateral (Zone II)	Usually explore	Usually do not explore
Pelvic (Zone III)	Explore	Do not explore

The Abbreviated Trauma Laparotomy (Damage Control)

When physiology is disrupted attempts at restoring anatomy are futile

In a small minority of patients with a critical physiological status time-consuming organ repair cannot be undertaken safely. A bailout procedure consisting of temporary control of bleeding and contamination is then indicated. *These cases can be recognized either by physiological criteria or by a complex pattern of anatomical injuries.* In the first setting, the presence of coagulopathy, hypothermia and acidosis – the *triad of death* – singly or in combination, are pointers to impending physiological exhaustion. In the second setting, the combination of severe and complex injuries (for example, a major vessel injury associated with a severe duodeno-pancreatic disruption) is recognized early as a precursor of major blood loss and a prolonged reconstructive procedure, in an unstable patient. In these circumstances, the surgeon may opt for expeditious control of the hemorrhage (usually by packing) and the simplest means of preventing further peritoneal contamination. Abdominal closure would then consist of rapid cutaneous approximation or is avoided all together. The patient is then transported to the surgical intensive care unit where secondary stabilization is undertaken over the next 24–48 hours. Delayed definitive organ repair and abdominal closure are effected only when secondary resuscitation has been achieved.

28 The Abdominal Compartment Syndrome

In surgery physiology is the king, anatomy the queen;
you can be the prince, but only provided you have the judgement...

At Thanksgiving – a national holiday here in the USA – many millions of Turkeys – also called "Thanksgivings Birds" – are tightly stuffed with various sorts of ingredients and served to the craving mouths of meat-loving Americans. Mind, however, that these large birds are stuffed post-mortem, not before. Imagine what would have happen to the poor bird, if tightly stuffed – into her abdomen, and alive – with your favorite sort of stuffing (mine would include chickpeas, garlic, wine-soaked bread, and thyme). First, the bird would stop flying and then gradually it would hypoventilate, collapse and die. Surely, you could attribute the death of the stuffed avis to bad lungs, old heart, toxins produced by the ingredients used in the stuffing and as always – you could blame the anesthetist. But frankly, there is a huge body of first grade scientific evidence, to prove beyond any doubt that the tragic outcome of your bird resulted from elevation of her intra-abdominal pressure (*IAP*), causing *intra-abdominal hypertension (IAHT)* which in turn leads to the *abdominal compartment syndrome (ACS)*.

Does Abdominal Compartment Syndrome (ACS) Exist?

A large body of knowledge supports the concept that elevated *IAP or IAHT* may impair physiology and organ function by producing the *abdominal compartment syndrome (ACS)*. Complex, adverse physiological consequences of increased IAP develop as it is transmitted onto adjacent spaces and cavities, decreasing cardiac output, restricting pulmonary ventilation, diminishing renal function and visceral perfusion, and increasing cerebrospinal pressure (Table 28.1 and Figure 28.1).

254   **Table 28.1.** Physiological consequences of intra-abdominal hypertension.

	Increased	Decreased	No change
mean blood pressure	–	–	X
heart rate	X	–	–
peak airway pressure	X	–	–
thoracic/pleural pressure	X	–	–
central venous pressure	X	–	–
pulmonary capillary wedge pressure	X	–	–
Inferior vena cava pressure	X	–	–
renal vein pressure	X	–	–
systemic vascular resistance	X	–	–
cardiac output	–	X	–
venous return	–	X	–
visceral blood flow	–	X	–
gastric mucosal pH	–	X	–
renal blood flow	–	X	–
glomerular filtration rate	–	X	–
cerebrospinal fluid pressure	X		–
abdominal wall compliance	–	X	–

At the bedside, IAP is best measured through the urinary bladder catheter connected into a manometer or a pressure transducer. In fact, all you need to measure IAP is a Foley catheter: disconnect it from the collecting tube; install 100 ml of saline into the bladder and elevate the now re-connected collecting tube perpendicular to the supine patient and his bed. The height of the urine column in the tube is the IAP in cm'-water (one cm water = 0.735 mmHg). A neurogenic or small contracted bladder may render the measurements invalid. Errors can also occur if the catheter is blocked or in the presence of a pelvic hematoma which may selectively compress the bladder. Because Trendelenburg positions (or its reverse) may affect intra-bladder pressures, accurate measurements are best achieved in the supine position.

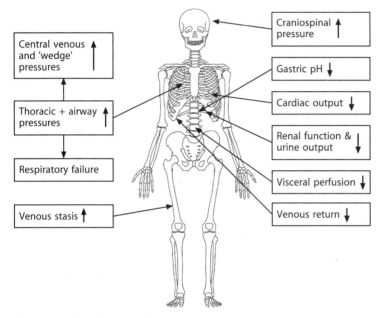

Fig. 28.1. The abdominal compartment syndrome

Deleterious Consequences of Raised IAP Appear Gradually

At pressures less than 10 mmHg cardiac output and blood pressure are normal but hepatic arterial blood flow falls significantly; IAP of 15 mmHg produces adverse cardiovascular, but easily compensable, changes; IAP of 20 mmHg may cause renal dysfunction and oliguria, and an increase to 40 mmHg induces anuria. In an individual patient, the effects of increased IAP are not isolated but usually superimposed on multiple underlying and co-existent factors, the most notable being hypovolemia, which aggravates the effects of increased IAP.

256   Why Didn't You Observe IAHT & ACS Before?

Because you did not know that this entity exists! Any increase in the volume of any of the contents of the abdomen or the retroperitoneum elevates IAP. Clinically significant elevation of IAP has been observed in a variety of contexts such as: postoperative intra-abdominal hemorrhage, after complicated abdominal vascular procedures or major operations such as hepatic transplantation, in association with severe abdominal trauma accompanied by visceral swelling, hematoma or the use of abdominal packs; severe peritonitis, use of pneumatic antishock garment and tense ascites in cirrhotic patients. Peritoneal insufflation during laparoscopic procedures is currently the most common (iatrogenic) cause of IAHT. Note that severe intestinal edema causing IAHT was described following massive fluid resuscitation for *extra-abdominal* trauma (Table 28.2).

Be aware that *morbid obesity* and *pregnancy* (chapter 25) *are "chronic" forms of IAHT*; various manifestations associated with such conditions (e.g. hypertension, pre-eclampsia) are attributed o IAHT. Note that *anything* can cause IAHT and ACS – irrespective of the ingredients used in the "stuffing" or its flavor. The "stuffing" can be even composed of feces:

> An elderly lady presented with poor peripheral perfusion, blood pressure of 70/40, and respiratory rate – 36/min. Her abdomen was very distended, diffusely tender with guarding. Rectal examination revealed a large amount of soft impacted feces. BUN and creatinine levels were 30mg% and 2mg%, respectively. Arterial blood gases showed a metabolic acidosis with pH of 7.1. Her IAP was 25 cm' water. She survived following a decompressive laparotomy and resection of the massively dilated and partially ischemic rectosigmoid.

Only a few years ago we would have described this patient as suffering from "septic shock" due to "colonic ischemia". We would have attributed the cardiovascular collapse and acidosis to the consequences of endo-

Table 28.2. Etiology of increased intra-abdominal pressure*

ACUTE	
I. Spontaneous	Peritonitis, intra-abdominal abscess, ileus, intestinal obstruction, ruptured abdominal aortic aneurysm, tension pneumoperitoneum, acute pancreatitis, mesenteric venous thrombosis
II. Postoperative	Postoperative peritonitis, paralytic ileus, acute gastric dilatation, intra-peritoneal hemorrhage
III. Posttraumatic	Intra/retro-peritoneal bleeding, post-resuscitation visceral edema
IV. Iatrogenic	Laparoscopic procedures, pneumatic anti-shock garment, abdominal packing, reduction of a massive parietal or diaphragmatic hernia, abdominal closure under excessive tension
CHRONIC	Ascites, large abdominal tumor, chronic ambulatory peritoneal dialysis, pregnancy, morbid obesity

*   The list below cannot be considered "complete" as any increase, of any etiology, in the volume of the intra-or retroperitoneal space will increase intra-abdominal pressure.

toxemic sepsis. But today it is clear to us that the mass- effect created by the extreme dilatation of the rectum produced severe IAHT, causing cardiovascular and respiratory collapse and renal dysfunction – representing a typical ACS. The latter, further decreased splanchnic perfusion, thus aggravating colorectal ischemia. Rectal dis-impaction and abdominal decompression rapidly reversed the adverse physiological manifestations of the abdominal hypertension. Being more aware that IAHT is a "real problem" and liberally measuring IAP, we recognize it with an increasing frequency in our daily clinical practice.

258 The Mechanisms Culminating in an ACS Are Usually Multiple

The typical scenario occurs in a multiple trauma or post emergency laparotomy patient who receives a large volume of fluid for resuscitation, causing an increase in interstitial fluid volume. The ensuing visceral and retroperitoneal edema is aggravated by shock-induced visceral ischemia and reperfusion edema, as well as by temporary mesenteric venous obstruction caused by surgical manipulation or the employment of hemostatic packs. The edematous abdominal wall is closed over the bulging abdominal contents under extreme tension.

The Clinical Syndrome

The clinical syndrome of ACS consists of:
• need for increased ventilatory pressure
• presence of decreased cardiac output
• decreased urinary output

– the above variables – present despite an apparently "normal" or increased cardiac filling pressures (Increased IAP, when "transmitted" to the thorax, proportionally elevates central venous pressure, pulmonary capillary wedge pressure, and right atrial pressure increase) in association with abdominal distention. Cardiovascular, respiratory and renal dysfunction becomes progressively difficult to manage unless IAP is reduced. Rarer consequences of ACS were described, such as intestinal ischemia following laparoscopic cholecystectomy or spinal cord infarction in the setting of IAHT following a perforation of a gastric ulcer.

When Should You Consider Abdominal Decompression?

The decision to decompress the abdomen should not be taken based on isolated measurements of IAP without taking into account the whole clinical picture. Early or mild physiological abnormalities caused by IAHT can be maneuvered by fluid administration or afterload reduction. Established ACS, however, mandates an emergency decompressive laparotomy, which, when performed in the well-resuscitated patient, promptly restores normal physiology. To prevent hemodynamic decompensation intra-vascular volume should be restored, oxygen delivery maximized, and hypothermia and coagulation defects corrected. Following decompression, the abdominal skin and fascial edges are left open using one of the temporary abdominal closure devises (TACD) described in chapter 37.

Prevention

In order to avoid IAHT & ACS, forceful closure of the abdomen in patients having massive retroperitoneal hematoma, visceral edema, severe intra-abdominal infection, or a need for hemostatic packing, should be avoided (chapter 29). Leaving the fascia open, closing only the skin with sutures or towel clips to protect the bulging viscera, has been recommended. Occasionally, however, only the skin closure may produce IAP of 50 mmHg or more. Certainly, leaving both fascia and skin unsutured offers maximal reduction in IAP but may result in fistula and evisceration. Bridging the fascial gap with prosthesis circumvents these problems (chapters 29,36,38,39).

260 Would Decompression Benefit Patients with only a Moderate IAHT?

That the "extreme" case of ACS as described above necessitates an urgent abdominal decompression is obvious. But what about a "less extreme" case? Would decompression benefit a postoperative patient in whom the moderately increased IAP of 20 mmHg is compensated by appropriate fluid and ventilatory therapy? We believe that the available evidence suggests that the detrimental effects of IAHT take place long before the manifestation of ACS become clinically evident just as nerve and muscle ischemia begins long before neuromuscular signs of the extremity compartment syndrome are evident. IAHT may cause gut mucosal acidosis at lower bladder pressures, long before the onset of clinical ACS. Uncorrected, it may lead to splanchnic hypoperfusion, distant organ failure and death. Prophylactic non-closure of the abdomen may facilitate the prevention, early recognition and treatment of IAHT and reduce these complications. It appears thus that also a "borderline" IAHT contributes to the overall morbidity but the benefit-risk ratio of abdominal decompression in such patients is not clear as yet.

In conclusion: IAHT is yet another factor to consider in the overall management of the emergency abdominal patient. It may be obvious – "crying" for abdominal decompression. More commonly, however, it is relatively silent but contributing to your patient's SIRS, organ dysfunction and death. So now you know better, you know that your patient is not a dead Turkey to be stuffed. Bon appetite!

Be aware of intra-abdominal hypertension as you are aware of arterial hypertension.
It is much more common and clinically relevant than you have suspected hitherto.

29 Abdominal Closure

Big continuous bites, with a monofilament and – above all
– avoiding tension – this is how to avoid dehiscence and herniation

Finally, it is time to get the" hell out of here". You were working all night and it is tempting to do so hastily. Impatience, however, is inadvisable since correct abdominal closure would protect the patient from abdominal wound dehiscence and yourself from a great humiliation ("everybody knows"), and later on, from the development of a hernia.

Yes, you are tired but before closing check again for hemostasis, ask if the swab count is OK – ask but trust nobody and feel around. See that the small bowel lies comfortably – covered with omentum if available. Are the drains inserted correctly – away from bowel? Now stop and think; ask your assistants: "did we forget to do something?" A jejunostomy tube for example (chapter 31).

Generally, an abdominal closure fails because of poor quality of the tissues, increased intra-abdominal pressure, faulty technique, or a combination of the aforementioned. Occasionally, a suture knot comes undone, but the commonest failure mode implies that the *tissue is torn, not the suture.* In order to achieve secure closure keep in mind (and hands) the following.

Principles of Closure

Suture Material

Use a non-absorbable (e.g. nylon or prolene) or "delayed" absorbable (e.g. PDS or maxon) monofilament suture. Rapidly absorbed material such as vicryl and dexon are still widely used even though their use is illogical in view of wound-repair kinetics. Those who fancy such suture

262   material produce the hernias for us to repair. Non – or slowly absorbable suture material, on the other hand, keeps the edges of wound together until its tensile strength "takes over". Monofilament sutures are advantageous because they "slide" better, inflicting less "saw-injury" to the tissues and, when used in the preferred continuous fashion, better distribute the tension along the length of the wound. The use of braided non-absorbable material (i.e. silk) is associated with chronic infected sinus formation and belongs, we hope, to the remote history.

"Mass Closure"

This is the preferred technique as documented in numerous studies. It has been popularized for the closure of midline incisions but is as effective for the closure of transverse – muscle cutting incisions. For the latter, however, many surgeons still prefer layered (posterior fascia-anterior fascia) closure.

"Mass closure" entails mono-layered suturing of *all* structures of the abdominal wall in a continuous manner to provide "one strong scar". The secret here is to take "large bites" of tissue, almost an inch away from the wound's edges; the bites should be closely spaced so not to create gaps greater than one cm'. Evade the common mistake of avoiding to include muscle with your fascial bites; this may look cosmetically appealing as the muscle is "hidden away" under the fascia, but does not produce the desired "mass scar". Not less important is the issue of the *correct tension* to be set on the suture. If you pull too tight on the suture the tissue is strangulated and necrosed; if you keep the suture too loose the wound edges gap. A suture length to wound length ratio of at least 1:3 will ensure a moderate but secure tension of closure. The corners of the incision are the Achilles heels of closure, especially the corner which is closed the last. Do not compromise the complete closure of the corner because you are afraid to injure the underlying bowel; there are good tricks to accomplish this endeavor – learn them from one of your mentors.

Do not harm the underlying bowel, which frequently bulges
towards your large needle. At the end of the operation the anesthetist
always swears to God that the patient is "maximally relaxed"; usually,
however, it is not so – make him relax the patient again – do not compromise. Protect the bowel by whichever instrument available, the best, in
our experience, being the commercially available rubber "fish" retractor.
The assistant's hand may be useful for this purpose but with all the
hepatitis and HIV around we do not find many volunteers willing to
offer a retracting hand.

We recommend the use of a "looped" number 1 PDS suture. It is
a slowly- absorbable monofilament, long enough to provide suture-
to-wound ration of 1:3. Threading the needle through the loop after the
first "bite" replaces the need for the "initial" knot.

The Subcutaneous Space

Now when the fascia is closed what to do with subcutis? Nothing! There
is no evidence that the so-called "dead space reduction" using subcutaneous fat approximation reduces wound complications. On the contrary;
subcutaneous sutures serve as a foreign body, strangulate viable fat
while not producing a more satisfactory wound. *Subcutaneous drains
increase* the rate of infection and are almost never indicated. Plain saline
irrigation of the subcutis has been shown useless, but use of topical antibiotics, (solution or powder) has been demonstrated to further decrease
wound infection rate in patients who already received systemic antibiotic
prophylaxis.

264   ## What About the Well Entrenched Ritual of 'Delayed Primary' or 'Secondary Closure' After Contaminated or Infected Laparotomies?

We believe that these techniques are only rarely indicated. In spite of surgeons' obsession with tradition, lessons learned years ago under certain circumstances are not necessarily true today. Thus, twenty years ago when antibiotic prophylaxis was given incorrectly, heavy silk sutures were buried in the fat, and rubber drains where mushrooming through each wound, the rate of infections developing in the primarily closed wounds was intolerable. Today, on the other hand, with proper surgical technique and modern antibiotic prophylaxis, primary suture of the wound can be undertaken uneventfully in the majority of the emergency laparotomy cases. When a wound infection develops it usually responds to local measures. Thus, leaving all contaminated/infected wounds gaping open – awaiting spontaneous or secondary closure, produces unnecessary physical and financial morbidity. We decide NOT to close the wounds very occasionally; usually in patients with gross, established purulent or fecal peritonitis, in patients planned for further re-operations or in the re-laparotomized abdomen. In the vast majority of patients we irrigate the subcutaneous tissues with antibiotics (after fascial closure) and close the skin with staples or interrupted sutures. An occasional wound infection is not a disaster and is simple to treat (chapter 40).

The High Risk Abdominal Closure

Classically, in patients with systemic (e.g. cancer) or local (e.g. abdominal distension) factors associated with, and predicting a high risk for wound dehiscence, *"retention"* sutures were and are still used by surgeons. Those heavy "through and through" interrupted sutures

take large bites through all abdominal-wall layers – including the skin –   265
preventing evisceration but not the occurrence of late hernia formation.

We do not find any use for the *classic "retention"* sutures, which also cut through the skin, producing parietal damage and ugly skin wounds and scars. Instead, we suggest that in selected high-risk closures, you place a few interrupted all layers "mass" sutures (excluding the skin) to take the tension off the continuous "mass" closure. Should the latter fail at any point the interrupted sutures would prevent separation of the fascial edges and evisceration.

The crucial consideration is, however, that *"retention"* (sutures) *together with abdominal distension, results in intra-abdominal hypertension.* Forceful closure under excessive tension may result in an abdominal compartment syndrome with its deleterious physiological consequences (chapter 28). Thus, when the fascia is destroyed as is often the case after multiple abdominal re-entries, or when closure may produce excessive intra-abdominal pressure *we suggest that you do not close the abdomen but cover it with a temporary abdominal closure device (TACD)* (chapters 28,36,37).

> In conclusion – remember:
> **Big continuous bites, with a monofilament**
> **and – above all – avoiding tension**
> **– this is how to avoid dehiscence and herniation**

30 Ruptured Abdominal Aneurysm

Abdominal pain and hypotension equals a ruptured AAA,
unless proven otherwise.

Urological and orthopedic wards are a cemetery for rupture AAA patients.

Presentation

The diagnosis of a leaking abdominal aortic aneurysm (AAA) is usually
not difficult to make. Typically the patient presents with a sudden onset
of acute lumbar backache, abdominal pain and collapse associated with
hypotension. On examination the presence of a pulsatile abdominal
mass confirms the diagnosis. In this situation the patient proceeds
directly to the operating room with a delay only to allow cross-matched
blood to become available if the patient is stable.

Atypical Presentation

Not infrequently, however, the diagnosis can be difficult to make. There
may be no history of collapse and the patient may be normotensive on
admission. The only clue may be non-specific back or abdominal pain.
A pulsatile mass may not be palpable. Ruptured AAA patients are
frequently obese; thinner patients tend to notice their AAA and present
early for an elective repair. A leaking AAA may be mislabeled as "ureteric
colic" but the absence of microscopic hematuria should alert one to the
possibility that a leaking aneurysm is responsible for the symptoms.
A high index of suspicion is important to prevent the diagnosis of a
leaking AAA being overlooked. In appropriate individuals, particularly
men in late middle age and old age, abdominal aneurysms should be
excluded by means of ultrasound or CT, if significant and unexplained
abdominal or back pain causes the patient to present acutely.

The Diagnostic Dilemma

A different diagnostic dilemma occurs in patients who are known to have aneurysms and who present with abdominal or back pain, which may or may not be related to the aneurysm. The difficulty here is that a small, contained, "herald" leak from an aneurysm might produce pain without any hemodynamic instability. Examination in these patients may be unhelpful in that the aneurysm may not be tender. These patients are at high risk of a further bleed from their aneurysm, which could be sudden and catastrophic. It is important therefore that they are identified appropriately and receive surgical treatment before a further possibly fatal bleed.

The difficulty of course is that such a patient might easily have another cause for their symptoms, for example mechanical backache, which is unrelated to the aneurysm. Here, an emergency operation is clearly not in the patient's best interests, particularly if his or her general health is poor. This dilemma, of operating without delay in patients who require it, yet avoiding operation in those in whom it is not necessary, is a difficult one, sometimes even for experienced clinicians to resolve. An emergency CT scan is indicated in this situation to delineate the AAA and the absence or presence of an associated leakage – usually into the retroperitoneum. In general, however, it is safer to err on the side of operating on too many rather than too few patients.

The Operation

It is impossible to fill a bucket which has a hole

A useful rule of thumb is that the chances of survival in a patient with a ruptured AAA are directly proportional to the blood pressure on admission. Shocked patients rarely survive; sure, they may come alive

out of the operation but usually do not leave hospital through the front   269
door. Consequently, it has been proposed that operating on shocked
ruptured AAA patient is a futile waste of resources. Another view is that
you should proceed with the operation unless the patient is clearly
"agonal" or known to suffer from an incurable disease. You may be able
to save the occasional patient and to gain additional experience, which
may help you to save the next patient. These issues of philosophy of
care are for the individual surgeon to resolve with his patients and their
families.

Once the diagnosis of aortic rupture has been established, or
strongly suspected, the patient should be taken to the operating theatre
without delay. Do not even bother with lines and i.v. fluids as what you
pour in will pour out, and increasing the blood pressure will increase the
bleeding.

"Prep and drape" for surgery while the anaesthetic team are
inserting the appropriate monitoring lines. Do not allow them, however,
to waste time by inserting unnecessary gimmicks such as the pulmonary
arterial catheter. Anesthesia should not be induced until you are ready to
make the skin incision; not infrequently the administration of muscle
relaxants, and the subsequent relaxation of the abdominal wall – abolishing
its tamponade effect, is sufficient to permit a further bleed from the
aneurysm with an immediate hemodynamic collapse.

Remember: Your Clamp on the Aorta Proximal to the Aneurysm Is More Important That Anything Else

- *Incision*: open the abdomen through a long mid-line incision
  extending from the xiphisternum to a point mid way between the
  umbilicus and the symphysis pubis. Occasionally, if the distal iliac
  arteries are to be approached, the incision must be extended
  distally. In most cases however, for the insertion of a simple aortic
  tube graft, an incision as described is adequate.

270 • *Proximal control*: upon entering the peritoneal cavity, the diagnosis
is confirmed rapidly by the presence of a large retroperitoneal
hematoma. The immediate priority is to obtain control of the aorta
proximal to the aneurysm. In the majority of patients who are stable
at this stage – with a contained retroperitoneal leak, there is time
to approach the aorta above the aneurysm just below the level of
the renal arteries. In patients who are unstable, rapid control of
aortic bleeding may be obtained by approaching the aorta just
under the diaphragm and temporarily applying a clamp there until
the infra-renal aorta can be dissected.

• *Subdiaphragmatic aortic control*: remember how you do a truncal
vagotomy? Just pretend you do it again. Incise the phrenoesophageal
ligament overlying the esophagus (feel the nasogastric tube under-
neath). With your index finger bluntly mobilize the esophagus to
the right; forget about hemostasis at this stage. Now feel the aorta
pulsating to the left of the esophagus, dissect with your index on
both sides of the aorta until you feel the spine – apply a straight
aortic clamps – pushing it "onto" the spine. Leave a few packs to
provide hemostasis and proceed as below.

• *Infra-renal aortic control*: returning to the matter of isolation of
the aortic neck, note that the main principle to be observed is not
to disturb the retroperitoneal hematoma while gaining control of
the proximal aorta. Once you enter the retroperitoneum at the
neck's level, dissect bluntly with your finger, or using the tip of the
suction apparatus, to identify and isolate the neck of the aneurysm.
Once the neck is identified carry on down both sides of the aorta
until the vertebral bodies are reached. Do not attempt to encircle
the aorta with a tape. Then apply a straight aortic clamp in an
anteroposterior direction with the tips of the jaws of the clamp
resting against the vertebral bodies. Placement of this clamp is
facilitated by placing the index and middle fingers of your non-
dominant hand on either side of the aorta so that the vertebral

bodies can be palpated. The jaws of the open clamp are then slid 271
along the backs of the fingers until the clamp lies in the appropriate
position. Now you can remove the subdiaphragmatic clamp.

- *Juxtarenal neck*: occasionally the aneurysm extends close to the
  origin of the renal arteries. If this is the case then the neck of the
  aneurysm will be obscured by the left renal vein, which may be
  stretched anteriorly. Care must be taken that the vein is not damaged.
  It may be divided to facilitate access to the aneurysm neck. This is
  done by very gently mobilizing the vein from the underlying aorta.
  It should be ligated securely as close to the vena cava as prudence
  permits. If this is done then the vein may be ligated with impunity
  and the kidney will not be endangered. Collateral venous drainage
  will take place via the adrenal and gonadal anastomoses.

- *How do you know that effective proximal control has been achieved?*
  Simple – the retroperitoneal hematoma stops pulsating. If it pul-
  sates your clamp is not properly placed. Re-apply it!

- *Distal control*: the next part of the dissection to identify the common
  iliac arteries is often more difficult. Under normal circumstances
  the pelvis is the site of accumulation of much of the retroperitoneal
  hematoma and the iliac arteries are buried within this. The arteries
  are difficult to locate not only because they are buried in hematoma
  but also because with the aorta clamped proximally, there is no
  pulsation to guide the operator. In most patients however the
  presence of atheroma in the vessels makes palpation in the depths
  of the hematoma possible. Again the use of the suction apparatus
  facilitates isolation of the iliac vessels. Otherwise, dig with your
  fingers within the hematoma and "fish" the iliacs out. As with the
  aorta, no attempt should be made to encircle the iliac vessels with
  tapes. This invariably produces damage to the iliac veins, which is
  a disaster. It is sufficient to clear the anterior and lateral aspects of
  the iliac vessels and apply clamps in an anteroposterior manner as
  before.

272 • *An alternative-balloon control*: after proximal control has been
        achieved and when the iliacs are immersed within a huge hematoma
        you may also rapidly open the aneurysm sac and shove two Foley
        or large Fogarty catheters into both iliacs – inflating the balloons
        to produce temporary distal control.
     • *Aortic replacement*: once the proximal and distal arterial tree is
        controlled, incise the aneurysm sac in a longitudinal fashion.
        Evacuate the clot and control back bleeding from any patent lumbar
        arteries and the inferior mesenteric artery with sutures within the
        aneurysm sac. A small self-retaining retractor placed within the
        aneurysm sac to retract its cut edges facilitates this and the next
        few stages of the procedure.

The proportion of patients in whom aortic replacement with a simple
tube graft can be achieved varies widely from surgeon to surgeon and
center to center. We believe that in the majority of patients insertion of a
tube graft can be achieved quite satisfactorily. The advantages of this are
that limited dissection in the pelvis minimizes the risk of damage to the
iliac veins and the autonomic nerves. Furthermore, there seems little
point in extending the length of what is already a challenging operation
by inserting a bifurcation graft unnecessarily. Obviously there are
situations where a tube graft is not acceptable: namely where the patient
has occlusive aorto-iliac disease; where the iliac arteries are also
significantly aneurysmal; or in some situations where the bifurcation is
widely splayed so that the orifices of the common iliac arteries are far
apart.

Take care when fashioning the aorta to receive the graft. The
longitudinal incision in the aortic sac should be terminated at both ends
by a transverse incision so that the incision becomes 'T' shaped at each
end. The limbs of the 'T' should not extend more than 50% of the
circumference of the normal aorta, either at the proximal or distal ends.

Suture the graft in place using monofilament 3-0 material so that a   273
parachute technique can be used. This allows you to visualize clearly the
placement of the individual posterior sutures. Large bites of the posterior
aortic wall should be taken because the tissues in this situation are often
very poor. Furthermore, leaks, which occur after completion of the
anastomosis, are notoriously difficult to repair if they are situated at the
back wall. Once the upper anastomosis has been completed, a clamp is
applied to the graft just below the anastomosis and the clamp on the
aorta then released. Assuming there are no significant leaks at the upper
end, attention is turned to the distal anastomosis. This is completed in a
similar fashion to the proximal anastomosis.

Back bleeding from the iliac vessels should be checked before the
distal anastomosis is completed. Likewise, the graft should be flushed
with saline and one or two "strokes" of the patient's own cardiac output
to clear it of thrombogenic junk. If there is no back bleeding it may be
necessary to pass balloon embolectomy catheters into the iliac systems
to check that there has been no intra-vascular thrombus formation.
Once the distal anastomosis has been completed and found to be secure,
the iliac clamps should be released individually allowing time for any
hypotension to recover before the second clamp is removed. It is helpful
to the anesthetic team if the surgeon indicates when the time is
approaching for removal of the clamps. This allows the anesthetists to be
well ahead with fluid replacement. Inadequate fluid replacement at this
stage will result in significant hypotension when the iliac clamps are
released.

A word about heparin: it is clearly not sensible to administer
systemic heparin prior to cross-clamping in patients who are bleeding to
death from an aortic rupture. In patients in whom surgery has been
carried out for suspected rupture however and in whom no rupture is
found at operation, then systemic heparinization according to the
surgeon's normal practice should be carried out. It is permissible however
to heparinize locally the iliac vessels once the aneurysm sac has been

274   opened and back-bleeding from the small vessels has been controlled. Heparinized saline may be flushed down each of the iliac vessels in turn before re-applying the iliac cross-clamps. No consensus on the need for this practice has been reached and in the vast majority of patients it appears to be unnecessary.

Abdominal closure: commonly, the large retroperitoneal hematoma in combination with visceral swelling – produced by shock, resuscitation, re-perfusion and exposure, produce severe intra-abdominal hypertension manifesting after the closure of the abdomen. Rather than closing under excessive tension use temporary abdominal closure as discussed in chapters 28 and 37, and come back to close the abdomen another day. Avoidance of abdominal compartment syndrome is crucial for survival in these physiologically compromised patients in whom any further derangement is like a straw breaking the camel's back.

In emergency operations for AAA simplicity of the operation is a key for survival: rapid and atraumatic control, avoidance of injury to large veins, tube graft, minimal blood loss, and rapid surgery.

Many patients who reach the operating table will survive the operation only to die at its aftermath, usually due to associated medical illnesses such as myocardial infarction. A successful outcome therefore requires excellent post-op ICU care as well as competent surgery. Having completed the operation you won only half of the battle.

In ruptured AAA the operation is commonly the beginning of the end with the end arriving postoperatively.

Section C:

After the Operation

31 Nutrition

God created man with a mouth,
a stomach and gut-not a TPN line

The relatively brief interval available to you to prepare an emergency abdominal patient for an operation does not allow for nutritional considerations. The latter, therefore, are raised during and after the operation. Towards the end of the laparotomy you should ponder whether there is a need to provide an *enteral* access to facilitate postoperative feeding. After the operation the issues to think about are how early, and by which route, the patient should be fed.

Starvation

Starvation results in a state of adaptation, in which, after hepatic glycogen stores are consumed in 24 to 48 hours, the liver synthesizes glucose, using amino acids derived from protein breakdown. This "auto-cannibalization" of functional protein stores is ameliorated, to some degree, by conversion to ketone metabolism of the two major "obligate" glucose users, the CNS and the kidney. Fat stores help by providing ketones and, through glycerol metabolism, adding a small amount of glucose. Injury, illness or operation, though, greatly increases the demand for glucose to answer the hyper-metabolic demands made by SIRS and to provide energy for wound repair and for the bone marrow and its offspring, the leukocytes. The end result, then, is the breakdown of protein leading to general debility, impaired reparative processes and immune function, respiratory muscle weakness that in turn may cause atelectasis, pneumonia, ventilator-dependence and death.

278   The need for nutritional support then, is based on:
- Your physical and laboratory assessment of the patient's *nutritional reserves*.
- An estimate of the *associated stress of the underlying illness*.
- An estimate of *time interval*, which will pass before the patient can resume a normal diet.

Assessment of Need for Nutritional Support

You must ask the patients how long they have felt sick and how much weight they lost, if any, in the weeks prior to the operation. You must also ask when they last ate. By looking at the person you can estimate what their ideal weight might be and make a guess-estimate regarding the percent which has been lost. (Your rule of thumb standard is the fabled "70 kilogram man.") *A loss of more than 10% are associated with a higher rate of complications and death after abdominal surgery.* This will give you the first two pieces of information necessary for decision-making:
- Percent weight loss and available reserves.
- Time since normal feeding was stopped.

Serum albumin level reflects the balance of synthesis and degradation of one of the products of hepatic metabolism. In the emergency setting, the albumin level will be the only laboratory parameter available to you to estimate *available reserves*. A level of <3 mg/dl is associated with a higher rate of complications and death in abdominal surgery.

The associated stress of illness may be roughly estimated as minimal, moderate or maximal. It is better, though, to characterize stress by the use of a physiologic scoring system which measures the severity of the acute illness-such as the APACHE II system (chapter 5). *An increased level of stress is associated with a higher rate of protein breakdown as well as complications and death in abdominal surgery.*

The third piece of information necessary for decision-making is 279 *the time interval, which will pass before the patient can resume a normal diet.* This estimate is based on the nature of the primary illness and the type of operation, which is required or has been performed. For example, a person with "simple" acute appendicitis will experience cessation of normal feeding for a period of 24 to 72 hours whereas a person with perforated diverticulitis with generalized peritonitis may experience cessation of feeding for a period of 10 to 14 days.

With the above information, then, you can decide which patient will be most likely to benefit from nutritional support.

- At one end of the spectrum the patient with *normal reserves* by history and examination, with *minimal to moderate associated stress*, and with *less than 7–10 days estimated before resumption of a normal diet*, is *unlikely* to benefit from nutritional support.
- At the other end of the spectrum the patient with *depleted available reserves, moderate to severe stress and with more than 7 to 10 days estimated before resumption of a normal diet*, is *likely* to benefit from nutritional support.

Enteral vs. Parenteral Nutrition

Nutritional support may be provided by *enteral* – through the alimentary tract or *parenteral*-intravenous – routes. The advantage of enteral nutrition is that it is less expensive, associated with fewer complications and, very likely, associated with improved immune function and decreased intestinal bacterial translocation. The advantage of parenteral nutrition is that it can be used when and if gastrointestinal tract is not functional. This is not controversial anymore: when the gut functions use it! Clearly, *enteral* feeding is safer, cheaper, and more physiologic than *parenteral* nutrition!

Enteral Nutrition

Tasty food given by mouth is the ideal. Oral feeding requires the cooperation of the patient, a normal swallowing mechanism and normal gastric motility. Unconscious and intubated patients, however, cannot swallow but the main problem is that following abdominal operations the stomach is lazier than the intestine. In other words, after laparotomy the small bowel recovers motility before the stomach. The gut is ready to absorb nutrients in the first postoperative day while the stomach may have delayed emptying for at least a few days (chapter 34). It is clear then, that when early postoperative feeding is deemed necessary, or when oral intake is inadequate, the food should be installed distally – beyond the esophagus and the stomach.

Routes

In general when the mouth is "not available" the following feeding routes are optional:

- *Nasogastric and nasoenteric.* The former is of course not usable when the stomach is not functioning. The later brings the nutrients directly into the craving duodenum and jejunum. Transnasal intubation – even with narrow – bore and soft tubes is uncomfortable, and may lead to nasal trauma, sinus infection and rarely to bronchial injury with inadvertent instillation of the feeding solution into the pleural space.
- *Gastrostomy and transgastric jeununal tube.* The feeding tube is operatively placed directly into the stomach, and/or through the pylorus into the jejunum. This is a surgical procedure, which violates the gastric wall. The chief complication, which is rare but potentially fatal, is leakage at the insertion site, around the tube, or into the peritoneal cavity.
- *Jejunostomy tube.* The feeding tube (or a catheter) is inserted directly into the proximal jejunum as discussed below.

Clearly, feeding directly into the jejunum – as opposed to gastric feeding –   281
is associated with a lesser risk of aspiration.

Should I Place a Jejunal Feeding Tube?

This is the question you should ask yourself at the end of the emergency
laparotomy. It is much more convenient to do it at this stage as opposed
to doing it postoperatively. You should consider the three questions
mentioned above: what is the likelihood that this patient will be eating
in 7–10 days?; is he malnourished or not?; and what is the magnitude of
illness?

A malnourished alcoholic patient who requires a total gastrectomy
with esophagojejunal anastomosis for massive upper gastrointestinal
bleeding – represents a classical indication for a jejunal (J) feeding tube.
A case of multi-trauma involving the thorax, pelvis and long bones, who
undergoes a laparotomy for hepatic injury, could also benefit from
immediate J-tube feedings. After a partial gastrectomy in a previously
well-nourished patent J-tube placement is not indicated – the potential
risks overriding the assumed benefits. Hey, you don't want to place
J tube in a patient who won't need it.

There Are Three Methods to Place the J Tube:

*   *Transnasally*-into the stomach from which you can manipulate it
    by palpation into the proximal jejunum. The advantage is that it
    does not require a gastrotomy or enterotomy; disadvantages are its
    nasal presence and risk of accidental dislodgment.
*   *Transgastric*-combined gastrostomy/jejunostomy tubes are available
    to allow gastric aspiration and jejunal feeding at the same time.
    Obviously gastrostomy has it's own complications – mainly leakage
    around the tube, leakage into the peritoneal cavity and abdominal
    wall cellulitis. A meticulous fixation of the stomach onto the
    abdominal wall is mandatory.

282   •   *Jejunostomy*-A 16 or larger French tube may be placed through a
        purse-string-controlled enterotomy and then suture-tunneled with
        serosa over the site of entry, extending 5 to 7 cm proximal ("Witzel
        technique"). Alternatively, a 12 or 14 gauge catheter may be "tunneled"
        into the jejunal lumen through a needle ("needle catheter tech-
        nique"). Both techniques require suture fixation of the bowel to the
        site of catheter entry in the abdominal wall in order to prevent
        intra-abdominal leakage of small bowel contents and feedings, if
        the tube is accidentally removed before an enterocutaneous tract is
        developed (in 7 to 10 days). Additional useful *"tricks"* are: fix the
        efferent and afferent portions of the loop to the abdominal wall to
        prevent kinking and obstruction at the site of the jejunostomy. The
        needle and catheter should pierce the abdominal wall obliquely – in
        a direct line with the bowel-wall "tunnel"; this will prevent kinking
        of the fine tube at the bowel-skin junction.

Continuous J-feeding may be instituted immediately following operation
in most cases. Diarrhea is a common problem requiring the adjustment
of the volume and concentration of the specific solution you prefer to
use. Be aware that nasojejunal tubes can be inserted across suture lines
and that feeding can be installed proximal to suture lines. Note also that
cases *of massive intestinal infarction were reported in critically ill
patients* receiving early postoperative jejunal feeding, possibly due to
increased metabolic demands on an already poorly perfused gut. Therefore, hold J feedings in unstable patients and those on vasopressors.
Small bowel ileus can prevent adequate J feeding – always think that
behind the non-resolving or re-appearing ileus may be a treatable cause
(chapter 34).

    You were probably approached by the manufactures of the new
"immuno-enhancing diets". Those are tube feeding formulas which
contain high concentrations of certain nutrients and are claimed to
"increase immunity", thus reducing postoperative infection rate. The

value of such expensive diets is questionable, as is the value of enteral
supplement with the amino-acid glutamine.

You can place a transnasal J-tube also after the operation – if indicated. This however is not easy and requires prolonged manipulations
under fluoroscopy. An alternative is to use a gastroscope, with a long
tube (e.g. nasobilliary) placed into the distal duodenum through the
biopsy channel of the scope and under vision. Clearly, intra-operative
placement is much easier. Please do not forget this option before closing
the abdomen.

Parenteral Nutritional

Patients who cannot eat and won't tolerate enteral feeding may need
a parenteral nutritional support, which comes in three "flavors":

- *Protein sparing hydration* takes advantage of the fact that 100 gm'
  of glucose a day suppresses hepatic gluconeogenesis by supplying
  much of the obligate glucose need seen in starvation. Two liters of
  dextrose 5% provide this amount of sugar. For the average "not so
  stressed" patient this is more than enough for the first seven
  postoperative days.
- *Peripheral parenteral nutrition (PPN)* contains amino acids in
  addition to a low concentration of glucose and may provide an additional protein-sparing effect when "stress" is added to starvation.
  It is useful in maintenance nutrition for an intermediate period
  of postoperative starvation – seven days to two weeks – as long as
  patients' peripheral veins last. This is so because PPN is a "vein
  destroyer" which requires a new venous access each day.
- *Total parenteral nutrition (TPN)* contains amino acids and a
  concentrated dextrose solution – to which a lipid solution is usually
  added – which can provide for an indefinite duration the total
  amount of nutritional requirements even in the face of maximal
  stress. As usual, bypassing physiology has a prize: TPN is associated

284

with a long list of mechanical-catheter related, infectious and metabolic complications and is rather expensive.

Measurement of Effectiveness of Nutritional Support

In the long term this can be calculated by observing the balance of protein synthesis and degradation reflected in serum proteins levels such as albumin (half-life 17 days) or transferrin (half-life 8 days). In the short term, particularly in the critically ill, nitrogen balance can be assessed by comparing the amount of nitrogen which is produced in the urine (24 hour urine specimen analyzed in the laboratory) with the amount of nitrogen which is given by nutritional support (written on the package).

So What Should You Do?

- First decide if nutritional support will be helpful by estimating *nutritional reserve, degree of stress and time interval to normal diet.*
- Hold off starting nutritional supplements until peri-operative IV fluid resuscitation has attenuated the effect of third -space fluid sequestration and the initial hypermetabolic, hyperglycemic physiologic picture has abated somewhat (usually within 24 hours).
- Calculate the nutritional requirement by formula (there is no shame in looking this up) or indirect calorimetry.
- Institute nutritional support.
- Measure the effectiveness of treatment by analysis of urinary nitrogen loss compared to the amount of nitrogen provided by the treatment.

"Routine" Oral Feeding

Fortunately, most of your emergency abdominal patients recover from the ileus, induced by the underlying disease and its surgical treatment, within a few days. Traditionally, resumption of oral intake was completed in stages. First there was the nasogastric (NG) tube, which was kept in situ for variable periods (chapter 33); then the tube was removed (according to the rules established by the local guru). After the patient professed the blessed sounds of flatus he was started on "sips", thereafter, gradually, being advanced from "clear fluids" to "mix fluids", "soft diet", until the great day when "normal diet" was allowed, usually indicating that discharge home is imminent. Is such a ritual or its variant still practiced in your environment? If yes you should know that its value is based on no evidence at all. In fact, there is scientific evidence to prove that starting the patient on solid feeds is as "safe" and tolerable as the staged method still practiced by many.

On the other side, there are surgeons, who maintain that a patient who devours a beefsteak a day after a colectomy is a testimony to their superb surgical skills. Also this attitude is wrong: what's the point to force-feed a patient who does not have an appetite. The physiological postoperative ileus of the gut is a response that must have some purpose; appetite and desire to eat return when intestinal motility recovers. Our approach is therefore to let the patient decide when to eat, what to eat and how much; he'll tell you when his stomach is ready for a steak!

Before we finish let us share with you a few truths:

- We know that *prolonged* starvation may be harmful but there is no proof that early re-feeding after surgery is beneficial.
- We know that when compared to postoperative TPN, enteral nutrition is associated with better results. However, in the absence of a non-fed control group in any of the studies, it is not clear whether enteral nutrition provides specific benefit or is it the TPN which is associated with an increased rate of complications.

286   • There is some evidence that early postoperative enteral nutrition may adversely affect respiratory function.

Summary

Abdominal catastrophes and their operative treatment are often complicated by compromised nutritional reserve, stress and a long interval before a normal diet is resumed. The result of these factors is the production of immunoparesis by "auto-cannibalization" of functional protein with associated morbidity and mortality. Nutritional support in selected patients may help to attenuate these effects. Driven by manufacturers, nutrition hospital services or "TPN teams", the current emphasis is to unnecessarily overfeed the surgical patient – provoking additional morbidity and costs. Artificial feeding is a double edge sword – be selective and cautious.

32 Postoperative Antibiotics

*No amount of postoperative antibiotics can compensate
for intra-operative mishaps and faulty technique,
or can abort postoperative suppuration necessitating drainage.*

The Issue

Perhaps an issue as apparently banal as postoperative antibiotics does
not deserve a separate chapter. Already in chapter 6, you read about
pre-operative antibiotics and in chapter 10 you were introduced to the
concepts of *contamination* and *infection* and their therapeutic implications. Why not just administer postoperative antibiotics routinely for any
emergency abdominal operation until the "patient is well"? This is in fact
a common practice in the surgical community in this country and around
the world: patients receive postoperative antibiotics for many days, many
of them are even discharged home on oral agents, "just in case". What is
wrong with this approach? Our aim is to convince you that indiscriminate
postoperative antimicrobial administration is *wrong* and to provide guidelines in order to approach this issue in a more rational way.

For a long time the topic of *duration* of administration has been
easily dismissed in the "official" literature, with the common laconic
recommendation that antibiotics should be continued until all signs of
infection, including fever and leukocytosis, subside, and the patient is
"clinically well". No evidence existed, however, to prove that indeed the
continuation of antibiotics along these lines could abort an infection-in-
evolution, or cure an existing one.

During the last decade, we learned that fever and white cell response
are part of the patient's inflammatory response to a variety of infective
and non-infective causes. We realized that sterile inflammation is common
after any operation, manifesting itself as a local inflammatory response

288   syndrome (LIRS), or a systemic one (SIRS) (chapter 38). Is there a need to administer antibiotics after the bacteria are already dead?

The evolving policy of *minimal antibiotic administration* represents a trend away from the use of postoperative therapeutic courses of "fixed" and often long duration; rather, you should attempt to stratify the infective processes into grades of risks, and to tailor the duration of administration to the severity of infection.

Duration of Postoperative Administration

We recommend the policy summarized in table 32.1. It is based on the following arguments:

- Conditions representing contamination do not require postoperative administration since the infectious source has been dealt with at operation; bacteria and adjuvants of infection are effectively removed by the host's defenses, supplemented by peritoneal toilet, and adequate tissue levels of pre-and intra-operative prophylactic antibiotics. By definition, *prophylaxis* should *not* be continued beyond the immediate operative phase.

- In processes limited to an organ amenable to excision (*"resectable infection"*), the residual bacterial inoculum is low. A postoperative antimicrobial course of 24 hours should suffice to sterilize the surrounding inflammatory reaction and deal with gut bacteria, which may have escaped across the necrotic bowel wall by translocation.

- *"Non-resectable infections"* with a significant spread beyond the confines of the involved organ should be stratified according to its severity. A therapeutic postoperative course of more than 5 days is usually not necessary. However, certain complex situations may need *extended* courses of postoperative antibiotics. A typical example is infected pancreatic necrosis where the nidus of infection is not readily eradicated in a once-for-all surgical procedure. Similarly,

Table 32.1. Duration of postoperative antibiotic therapy   289

Contamination: No postoperative antibiotics
- Gastroduodenal peptic perforations operated within 12 hours
- Traumatic enteric perforations operated with 12 hours
- Peritoneal contamination with bowel contents during elective or emergency procedures
- Appendectomy for early or phlegmonous appendicitis
- Cholecystectomy for early or phlegmonous cholecystitis

Resectable infection: 24-hour postoperative antibiotic course
- Appendectomy for gangrenous appendicitis
- Cholecystectomy for gangrenous cholecystitis
- Bowel resection for ischemic or strangulated necrotic bowel without frank perforation

"Mild" Infection: 48-hours postoperative antibiotic course
- Intra-abdominal infection from diverse sources with localized pus formation
- "Late" (more than 12 hours) traumatic bowel lacerations and gastroduodenal perforation with no established intra-abdominal infection

"Moderate" Infection: up to 5 days of postoperative antibiotics
   Diffuse, established intra-abdominal infection from any source

"Severe" Infection-more than 5 days of postoperative antibiotics
- Severe intra-abdominal infection with a source not easily controllable (e.g. infected pancreatic necrosis)
- Postoperative intra-abdominal infection

patients with postoperative peritonitis, where the control of the source of infection is questionable, should be considered for prolonged antibiotic therapy.

It should be quite clear that the commonplace, blind, extended antibiotic administration, for as long as fever or leukocytosis are present, should be abandoned. Pyrexia and white cell response represent usually a sterile,

290   peritoneal (LIRS) or systemic (SIRS), cytokine-mediated, inflammatory response; admittedly, they, less commonly, indicate the presence of a focus of persistent or recurrent infection. The former situation is self-limited and resolves without antibiotics. The latter represents usually suppurative infection, which should be treated by drainage of the intra-abdominal abscess (chapter 35) or the infected wound (chapter 40). Antibiotic treatment can neither prevent nor treat suppurative infection; it may only succeed in masking it.

By now you should understand that the persistence of inflammation beyond the appropriate therapeutic course is not an indication to continue, re-start or change antibiotics. What should be avoided is complacent reliance on the advice of the average infectious disease (ID) specialist; this can only lead to an expensive and often unnecessary diagnostic work-up and, even more alarmingly, to the prescribing of the latest antibiotic agent on the market. What should instead be done is, first, to stop the antibiotics. The fever will subside spontaneously in most patients, within a day or two, with little more than chest physiotherapy. At the same time, a directed search is undertaken for a treatable source of intra-or extraperitoneal infection. Surgeons are best placed to anticipate complications in their patients, and this is what is meant by a directed search: a search that is conducted with the full knowledge of the patient's initial disease process, the operative findings and the natural history of the surgical disease; in brief, a corpus of information that usually eludes the ID specialist.

We hope that you realize that unnecessary antibiotics are wrong because anything unnecessary in medicine is "bad medicine". In addition, the price to be paid is high, not only financially. Antibiotics are associated with patient-specific adverse effects (the list is long, think of the gravity of *C. difficile* colitis) and ecological repercussions such as drug-resistant nosocomial infections in your hospital.

Are you convinced?

33 Postoperative Care

As long as the abdomen is open you control it.
Once closed it controls you.

The long operation is finished, leaving you to savor the sweet postoperative "high" and elation. But soon, when your serum level of endorphins declines, you start worrying about the outcome. And worry you must, for the cocksure, macho attitude is a recipe for disasters. We do not intend to bring here a detailed discussion of postoperative care or to write a new surgical intensive care manual. We only wish to share with you a few basic aspects, which may be forgotten, drowned in a sea of fancy technology and gimmicks. The following are a few practical "commandments" for postoperative care:

1. Prevent "Guilt-Worry". Always ask yourself, before closing the abdomen: "am I totally satisfied with my procedure?" Don't silence the little inner voice that informs you that the anastomosis is somewhat dusky. You must be absolutely convinced, at this stage, that you have done the best that your patient deserves. If not, swallow your pride, do it again, or call for help. Hiding a potential problem will not solve it. And you will go back to sleep so much better.

2. Know Your Patient. This is no joke! How often do we encounter a postoperative patient looked after by someone who has no clue about the patient's pre and intra-operative details? Mistakes in management are more commonly done by those who "temporarily adopt" the case. Once you operate on a patient he/she is yours! "Shared responsibility" means that no one is responsible!

3. Touch-Examine Your Patient. Not only from the foot of the bed. Examining the chart or the ICU monitor is not enough. Look at the patient, smell and palpate him at least once a day. Wouldn't it be embarrassing to load your patient with IV antibiotics or CT scan his abdomen, while an unsuspected abscess is cooking under the wound dressing, begging to be simply drained at the bedside?

4. Treat the Pain.   You know the different drugs, and their modes of administration. Sure, you always prescribe postoperative analgesia, but ordering is not nearly enough. Most randomly questioned postoperative patients complain that they are under-treated for pain. Nurses tend to be stingy with analgesia. You are the man on the spot; see that your patient does not suffer unnecessarily.

5. Do Not "Crucify" Your Patient in the Horizontal Position.   Typically the patient is 'crucified' horizontally by the excessive use of *spaghetti* of monitoring cables, nasogastric tube, venous lines, drains, and urinary catheters. Free the patient from this paraphernalia as soon as possible; the nurses won't do it without your order. The earlier your patient is out of bed, sitting or walking about, the faster he will be going home. Conversely, keeping the patient in the supine position increases the incidence of atelectasis/pneumonia, deep vein thrombosis, decubitus ulcers, and prolongs paralytic ileus, all adding fuel to the inflammatory fire of SIRS.

6. Decrease the Plastic and Rubber Load.   Monitoring functions as an early warning system to detect physiological disturbances so that prompt corrective therapy could be instituted. The invasiveness of monitoring employed in the individual patient should be proportionate to the severity of disease: "*The sicker the patient, the greater number of monitoring tubes used, the less likely is survival*".

Complete discussion of the continuously growing number of monitoring
methods available today is beyond the scope of this chapter. However,
please note:

- In order to be able to respond to monitoring-generated warning
  signs you must fully understand the technology being employed.
  You should be able to distinguish between real acute physiological
  changes versus electrical or mechanical artifacts of observation.
- Understand that all methods of monitoring are liable to a myriad
  of potential errors, specific to the technique or caused by patient-
  related variables. Alertness and sound clinical judgment are
  paramount!
- Due to improving technology, monitoring is becoming more and
  more sophisticated (and expensive). Furthermore, monitoring
  techniques are responsible for a significant number of iatrogenic
  complications in the SICU. Use monitoring discriminatingly and
  do not succumb to the *Everest Syndrome*: *"I climb it because it is
  there"*. Before embarking on invasive monitoring ask yourself: *does
  this patient really need it?* Remember there are safer and cheaper
  alternatives to invasive monitoring: for example, in a stable patient,
  remove the arterial line, as the BP can be measured with a conventional sphingomanometer, PO2 transcutaneously, and blood tests
  drawn through phlebotomy. Each time you see your patient ask
  yourself which of the following can be removed: nasogastric tube,
  Swan Ganz catheter, central venous line, arterial line, peripheral
  venous line, Foley's catheter.

Nasogastric Tubes. Prolonged postoperative NG decompression to combat
gastric and intestinal ileus is a common baseless ritual. The concept that
the NG tube "protects" distally-placed bowel anastomosis is ridiculous as
liters of juices are secreted each day below the decompressed stomach.
Nasogastric tubes are extremely irritating to the patient, interfere with
breathing, cause esophageal erosions and promote gastroesophageal

294   reflux. Traditionally, surgeons keep the tube until the daily output drops below a certain volume (e.g. 400-ml); such a policy often results in unnecessary torture. It has been repeatedly demonstrated that most post-laparotomy patients do not need nasogastric decompression, not even following upper GI procedures, or need it for a day or two at most. In fully conscious patients, who are able to protect their airway from aspiration, NG tubes can be safely used selectively. Following an emergency abdominal operation, nasogastric decompression is compulsory though, in mechanically ventilated patients, in obtunded patients, and after operations for intestinal obstruction. In all other cases, consider removing the NG tube on the morning after surgery.

Drains. Despite the widely publicized dictum that it is impossible to effectively drain the free peritoneal cavity, drains are still commonly used and misused (chapter 10). In addition to the false sense of security and reassurance they provide, drains can erode into intestine or blood vessels and promote infective complications. We suggest that you limit the use of drains to the evacuation of an established abscess, to allow escape of potential visceral secretions (e.g. biliary, pancreatic) and to establish a controlled intestinal fistula when the bowel cannot be exteriorized. Passive, open-system drainage offers bi-directional route for microorganisms and should be avoided. Use only active, closed-system drainage systems, placed away from the viscera. The placing of a drain close to an anastomosis in the belief that a possible leak will result in a fistula rather than in peritonitis is a long-enduring dogma; drains have been shown to contribute to the dehiscence of a suture line. A policy like "I always drain my colonic anastomoses for 7 days" belongs to the dark ages of surgical practice. Remove drains as soon as they have fulfilled their purpose.

7. Obtain Postoperative Tests Selectively. The performance of *unnecessary* diagnostic procedures or *interpretative* errors in *indicated* diagnostic procedures commonly result in *false-positive* findings, leading, in turn, to an increasingly invasive escalation of diagnostic or therapeutic measures. Added morbidity is the invariable price.

8. Realize That the Problem Usually Lies at the Operative Site. The cause of fever or 'septic state' in the surgical patient is usually at the *primary site of operation unless proven otherwise.* Do not become a "surgical ostrich" by treating your patient for "pneumonia" while he is slowly sinking in multiple organ failure from an intra-abdominal abscess.

9. Temperature Is Not a Disease: Do Not Treat It as Such. Postoperative fever represents the patient's inflammatory response (SIRS) to different insults including infection as well as surgical trauma, atelectasis, transfusion and others. SIRS does not always mean sepsis (sepsis=SIRS + infection). Therefore, fever should not be treated automatically with antibiotics. It also should not be treated symptomatically with anti-pyretics as the febrile response may be beneficial to the host's defenses. The absolute level of temperature is of less importance than its trend.

10. Avoid Poisoning Your Patient With Antibiotics; Tailor Antibiotic Administration to the Patient. Avoid the common practice of administering antibiotics for as long as the patient is in the hospital and beyond. (chapter 32).

11. Be Frugal with Blood-Products Transfusions. Generally, the amount of transfused blood or derived products inversely and independently correlates with the outcome of the acute surgical disease. Donated blood is immunosuppressive and is associated with an increased risk of infection, sepsis and organ failure, not to mention the other well-known hazards. Transfuse your patient only if absolutely necessary. A patient requiring only one unit of blood does not require any at all. For the vast majority of patients, a hematocrit of 30% is more than satisfactory.

12. Do Not Starve or Over-Feed Your Patient; Use the Enteral Route Whenever Possible. (chapter 31).

13. Recognize and Treat Intra-abdominal Hypertension. (chapter 28).

14. Prevent Deep Vein Thrombosis (DVT) and Pulmonary Embolism. It is easy to forget DVT prophylaxis in the pre-operative chaos of emergency surgery. As a pilot goes over a checklist prior to any flight – you should be the one to inject the subcut heparin and/or to place the anti-DVT pneumatic device – *before* the operation. DVT prophylaxis should be continued postoperatively as long as the patient continues to be high risk for thrombosis.

15. Be the Leader and Take Responsibility. Many people tend to dance around your postoperative patient, giving consults and advice. But remember – this is not their patient, it is yours (chapter 4). At the Mortality and Morbidity Meeting (or in court), the others will say: "I just gave a consult" (chapter 42). The ultimate responsibility for all aspects of your patient's management falls squarely in your hands. Know when you need help and request it, preferably from one of your mentors. Solicits advice judiciously and apply it selectively. Relinquishing blindly the care of your postoperative patient to anesthesiologists, medical intensivists, or other modern "experts" may be a recipe for disasters.

> **– Avoid "consultantorrhea" which may adversely affect survival**

34 Postoperative Ileus Versus Intestinal Obstruction

The postoperative fart is the best music to the surgeon's ears ...

Five days ago you removed this patient's perforated appendix (chapter 22); you gave him antibiotics for 2–3 days (chapter 32) and by today you expected him to eat (chapter 31) and go home. Instead, your patient lies in bed with a long face and a distended abdomen, vomiting bile from time to time. What is the problem?

Definitions and Mechanisms

The term *ileus* as used in this book, and in daily practice, signifies a "paralytic ileus" – the opposite from mechanical ileus, which is a synonym for intestinal obstruction. In essence, the later consists of a mechanical stoppage to the normal transit along the intestine whereas the former denotes hindered transit because the intestines are "lazy".

In previous chapters (2 & 17) you noted that ileus of the small bowel, colon or both, can be secondary to numerous intra-abdominal (e.g. acute appendicitis) retroperitoneal (e.g. hematoma) or extra-abdominal (e.g. hypokalemia) causes, which adversely affects normal intestinal motility. Following abdominal operations, however, ileus is a "normal" phenomenon – it's magnitude directly proportional to the magnitude of the operation. In general, the more you do within the abdomen, the more you "manipulate" – the more pronounced will be the postoperative ileus.

Ileus

Unlike mechanical intestinal obstruction, which involves a segment of the small or large bowel, postoperative ileus concerns the whole length of the gut – from the stomach to the rectum. As mentioned in chapter 31, physiological postoperative ileus resolves gradually. The small bowel resumes activity almost immediately, followed, a day or so later, by the stomach, and then the colon, being the laziest, is the last to start moving.

The magnitude of the postoperative ileus correlates to some extent with that of the operation performed and the specific underlying condition. Major dissections, prolonged intestinal displacement and exposure, denuded and inflamed peritoneum, residual intra or retroperitoneal pus or clots, are associated with a prolonged ileus. Thus, for example, after simple appendectomy for non-perforated appendicitis the ileus is almost non-existing, while after a laparotomy for a ruptured AAA (chapter 30) expect the ileus to be prolonged. Common postoperative factors, which can aggravate ileus, are the administration of opiates and electrolyte imbalance. While the "physiological" postoperative ileus is "diffuse", ileus due to complications may be "local". A classical example of a local ileus is a postoperative abscess (chapter 35) which may "paralyze" an adjacent segment of bowel.

Early Postoperative Mechanical Intestinal Obstruction

You became familiar with small bowel obstruction (SBO) in chapter 17. Early postoperative SBO is defined as one developing immediately after the operation or within two weeks. Two primary mechanisms are responsible: *adhesions* and *internal hernia*.

Early post-laparotomy *adhesions* are immature, inflammatory, poor in collagen – thus "soft", and vascular. Such characteristics indicate that early adhesions may resolve spontaneously and that its surgical lysis may

be difficult and "bloody". Postoperative adhesions may be diffuse, involving   299
the whole length of the small bowel in multiple sites, as occasionally seen
following extensive lysis of adhesion for SBO (chapter 17). Localized obstructing adhesions may also develop at the operative site with the bowel
adherent, for instance, to an exposed Marlex mesh or a raw peritoneal
surface. The operation also may create new potential spaces into which
the bowel can herniate to be obstructed – forming *internal hernias.*
Typical examples are the partially closed pelvis after abdomino-perineal
resection, or the space behind an emerging colostomy. The narrower the
opening into the space – the more likely is the bowel to be trapped.

Diagnosis

*Failure of your patient to eat, fart or evacuate his bowel within 5 days after
a laparotomy signifies a persistent ileus.* The abdomen is usually distended
and silent to auscultation. Plain abdominal X- ray typically discloses a
significant gaseous distension of both the small bowel and the colon
(chapter 3). The diagnosis of SBO in the recently operated abdomen is
much subtler. Textbooks teach you that on abdominal auscultation ileus
is silent and SBO noisy – this may be theoretically true but almost impossible to assess in the recently operated upon belly. If your patient has
already passed flatus or defecated and then ceases to manifest these
comforting features, SBO is the most likely diagnosis. *The truth is that in
most instances the patient will improve spontaneously without you ever
knowing whether it was a SBO or "just" an ileus.*

   The natural tendency of the operating surgeon is to attribute the
"failure to progress" to an ileus rather than SBO and to procrastinate.
Procrastination is not a good idea, however. A distended and non-eating
patient is prone to the iatrogenic hazards of NG tube, IV lines, parenteral
nutrition, and bed rest (chapter 33). Be active and proceed with diagnostic
steps in parallel to therapy.

300   **Management**

Pass a NG tube – if not already in situ – to decompress the stomach, prevent aerophagia, relieve nausea and vomiting, and measure gastric residue. Carefully search and correct, if present, potential causes of prolonged ileus:

- Opiates are the most common promoters of ileus; pain should be controlled but not excessively and for too long.
- Measure and correct electrolyte imbalances.
- Consider and exclude the possibility that an intra-abdominal complication is the cause of the ileus or SBO. A hematoma, an abscess, an anastomotic leak, postoperative pancreatitis, postoperative acalculus cholecystitis – all can produce ileus or mimic SBO.
- Significant hypoalbuminemia leads to generalized edema – involving the bowel too. Edematous and swollen bowel does not move well; this is called *hypoalbuminemic entropathy* and should be considered.

Practically speaking if on the fifth post-laparotomy day your patient still presents features of ileus/SBO we recommend a plain abdominal X ray to assess the gas pattern (chapter 3). If the latter suggests an ileus or SBO a *gastrografin challenge* as described in chapter 17 may be useful in relieving both conditions.

Failure of the gastrografin to arrive at the colon denotes a SBO. In the early postoperative phase this is not an indication for a laparotomy. Intestinal strangulation almost never occurs in this situation and spontaneous resolution is common. *Resolution of SBO, however, rarely occurs beyond the tenth postoperative day.*

When the clinical picture suggests one of the above mentioned intra-abdominal causes of persistent ileus – an abdominal CT is indicated to pin-point the problem and, at times, to guide treatment (chapters 35, 37 & 39).

In the absence of intra-or extra-abdominal causes for ileus, and
when the "ileus" does not respond to the gastrografin challenge, the
diagnosis is SBO. Do not rush to re-operate; treat conservatively while
providing nutritional support (chapter 31). Lack of resolution beyond
10–14 days is an indication for re-laparotomy – which in itself may be
difficult and hazardous because of the typical early dense and vascular
adhesions cementing the bowel at many points.

Prevention

It is imperative to emphasize that you can, and ought to, prevent postoperative ileus or SBO by sound operative technique and attention to details.
Gentle dissection and handling of tissues, careful hemostasis to avoid
hematoma formation, leaving as little foreign bodies as possible, not
denuding the peritoneum unnecessarily, not creating orifices for internal
hernias, and not catching loops of bowel during abdominal closure, are
self explanatory essentials.

Specific Problems

The various primary operations may result in different and specific types
of postoperative obstruction and ileus.

Anastomotic Obstruction

A bowel anastomosis at any level may cause early postoperative upper
gastrointestinal, small bowel or colonic obstruction. Faulty technique
(chapter 11) is usually the cause. A self-limiting "mini" anastomotic leak
is often responsible but under diagnosed. Diagnosis is reached with
a contrast study – please-water-soluble! Most such early postoperative

302   anastomotic obstructions are "soft" and edematous – resolving spontaneously within a week or two. Do not rush to re-operate; a gentle passage
of an endoscope – if accessible – may confirm the diagnosis and "dilate"
the lumen.

Delayed Gastric Emptying

Often the stomach fails to empty following a partial gastrectomy or
a gastro-jejunostomy for any indication. This is more common when a
vagotomy has been performed or when a Roux-en Y loop has been constructed. At gastrografin study the contrast persistently sits in the stomach.
The differential diagnosis is between a gastric ileus (gastroparesis) and
mechanical obstruction at the gastro-jejunostomy or below it. A complete discussion of the various post-gastrectomy syndromes is beyond the
scope of this volume but remember this fundamental principle: *postoperative gastric paresis is self limited* – it will always resolve spontaneously
but may take as long as 6 weeks to do so. Exclude mechanical stomal
obstruction with an endoscope or contrast study and then treat conservatively with NG suction, nutritional support – try to pass a feeding tube
distal to the stomach (chapter 31). Parenteral *erythromycin* has been
shown to enhance gastric motility. Resist the temptation to re-operate
for gastric paresis for it will eventually resolve while re-operation may
only make things worse.

Summary

Exclude and treat causes of persistent ileus, treat SBO conservatively as
long as indicated, think about specific causes of SBO (e.g. herniation at a
laparoscopic trocar site) and re-operate when necessary. In most instances
ileus/SBO will resolve spontaneously.

35 Intra-abdominal Abscesses

"Signs of pus somewhere, signs of pus nowhere else,
signs of pus there – under the diaphragm".
This was 100% true when I was a student,
50% true when I was a resident. Today it is irrelevant...

The contents of this chapter could have been summarized in a sentence: an abscess is a pus-containing, confined structure, which requires to be drained by whichever means available at your disposition. We believe, however, that you want us to elaborate further.

Abscesses may develop anywhere within the abdomen, resulting from a myriad of conditions. Specific types such as the peri-appendicular or diverticular abscesses (chapters 22 & 23) are covered elsewhere in this book; this chapter will introduce you with general concepts – with emphasis of what probably is the commonest abscess in your practice – the *postoperative abscess.*

Definition and Significance

Erroneously, the term intra-abdominal abscess has been used – and still is – as a synonym with secondary peritonitis (chapter 10). This is not true as abscesses develop thanks to effective host defenses and represent a relatively successful outcome of peritonitis. *To be termed an abscess, the confined structure has to be walled off by an inflammatory wall and possess a viscous interior.* In contrary, free-flowing, contaminated or infected peritoneal fluid or loculated collections, which are deprived of a wall, represent a phase in the spectrum – continuum of peritoneal contamination/infection and not an abscess.

Classification & Pathogenesis

The immense spectrum of intra-abdominal abscesses makes its classification complex (table 35.1). But practically, abscesses are *visceral* (e.g.
hepatic or splenic) or *non-visceral* (e.g. subphrenic, pelvic), *intraperitoneal*
or *extra-peritoneal*. *Non-visceral* abscesses arise following the resolution
of diffuse peritonitis during which loculated areas of infection and suppuration are "walled off" and persist; or after a perforation of a viscus,
which is effectively localized by peritoneal defenses. *Visceral abscesses*
are caused by hematogenous or lymphatic dissemination of bacteria to a
parenchymatous viscus. Retroperitoneal abscesses may result from a
perforation of a hollow viscus into the retroperitoneum as well as by
hematogenous or lymphatic spread. Another distinction is between the
postoperative abscess – for the development of which we surgeons feel
responsible – and *spontaneous abscesses*, unassociated with a previous

Table 35.1. Classification of abdominal abscesses

Classification	Examples
Visceral vs. non-visceral	Hepatic vs. subphrenic
Primary vs. secondary	Splenic vs. appendiceal
Spontaneous vs. postoperative	Diverticular vs. peri-anastomotic
Intra-peritoneal vs. retroperitoneal	Tubo-ovarian vs. psoas
Simple vs. *complex	*Complex: • multiple (liver) • multiloculated • communication with bowel (leaking anastomosis) • associated with necrotic tissue (pancreatic) • associated with cancer
Anatomical	Subphrenic, subhepatic, lesser sac, paracolic, pelvic, interloop, perinephric, psoas

operation. A further clinically significant separation is between *simple*
abscesses and *complex abscesses*, (e.g. multiple, mutiloculated, associated
with tissue necrosis, enteric communication or tumor) which require a
more aggressive therapy and carry poorer prognosis. The *anatomical
classification*, based on the specific anatomical location of abscess –
which typically develops in one of the few constant potential spaces –
has diminished in significance since the availability of modern imaging
and percutaneous drainage techniques.

Note that abscesses signify an *intermediate* natural outcome of
contamination/infection. On the one end of spectrum infection persists,
spreads and kills, on the other end, the process is entirely cleared by
host's defenses-assisted by your therapy. Abscesses lies in the no man
land, where the peritoneal defenses are only partially effective – being
disturbed by an overwhelming number of bacteria, micro -environmental
hypoxemia or acidosis, and adjutants of infections such as necrotic debris,
hemoglobin, fibrin and barium sulfate. An abdominal abscess won't kill
your patient immediately but if neglected – undrained, it becomes
gradually lethal, unless spontaneous drainage ensues.

Microbiology

Generally speaking the bacteriology of abdominal abscesses is polymicrobial.
Abscesses which develop in the aftermath of secondary peritonitis (e.g.
appendiceal or diverticular abscess) possess the mixed aerobic-anaerobic
flora of secondary peritonitis (chapters 6 & 10). It appears that while endotoxin
generating facultative anaerobes such as *E.coli,* are responsible for the phase
of acute peritonitis, the obligate anaerobes, such as *Bacteroides fragilis,*
are responsible for late abscess formation. These bacteria act in *synergy*:
both are necessary to produce an abscess and the obligate anaerobe can
increase the lethality of an otherwise non- lethal inoculum of the facultative
micro-organism. The vast majority of visceral abscesses (e.g. hepatic and

306   splenic) are polymicrobial-aerobic, anaerobic, Gram negative and positive. This is also true for retroperitoneal abscesses. Primary abscesses, such as the psoas one, are often mono–bacterial, with *Staphylococci* predominating. Postoperative abscesses are often characterized by the flora typical of tertiary peritonitis – representing superinfection with yeasts and other opportunists (chapter 38). The low virulence of these organisms, which represent a marker of tertiary peritonitis, and not its cause, reflects the global immunodepression of the affected patients.

Clinical Features

Clinical presentation of abdominal abscesses is as heterogeneous and multifaceted as the abscesses themselves. The spectrum is vast; systemic repercussions of the infection vary between a frank septic shock to nothing at all when suppressed by immunoparesis and antibiotics. Locally the abscess may be felt through the abdominal wall, the rectum or vagina; in most instances however it remains physically occult. In our modern times, when any fever is an alleged indication for antibiotics, most abscesses are initially "partially treated" or "masked" – presenting as a systemic inflammatory response syndrome (SIRS) with or without multi-organ dysfunction (chapter 38). Ileus is another not uncommon presentation of abdominal abscess; in the postoperative situation it is an "ileus which fails to resolve" (chapter 34).

Diagnosis

Life has become simple! Modern abdominal imaging has revolutionized the diagnosis of abdominal abscesses. Yes, you still need to suspect the abscess and carefully examine your patient but the definitive diagnosis (and usually the treatment) depends of imaging techniques. Computed tomography (CT), ultrasound (US) and various radioisotope-scanning techniques are available. Which is the best?

Radioisotope scanning with whichever radiolabeled material does not provide any anatomical data beyond localization of an inflammatory site; they are not accurate enough to permit percutaneous (PC) drainage. The usefulness of these methods is limited therefore to the continuous survival of nuclear medicine units and an excuse to publish papers. Practically, these tests have no role at all. Both US and CT provide good anatomical definition including the abscess's site, size and structure; both can guide PC drainage. US is portable, cheaper, and more accurate at detecting abscesses in the right upper abdomen and pelvis. It is, however, extremely operator dependent. We – surgeons – are better trained to read CT scans than US; hence we prefer the CT which allows us to visualize the entire abdomen, independently assessing the anatomy of the abscess, and plan its optimal management. *CT-intravenously, and intra-luminaly contrast-enhanced is also helpful in classifying the abscess either as simple or complex* (table 35.1).

It appears that performing multiple tests – adding a CT to an US – is not productive. Do understand that CT or US scanning during the first postoperative week is futile because neither technique can distinguish between a sterile fluid collection (e.g. residual lavage fluid), an infected fluid collection or a frank abscess. The best and only way to document the infective nature of the visualized fluid is a *diagnostic aspiration* – subjecting the aspirate for a Gram stain and culture. CT features, which however may hint that one deals with a proper abscess, are a contrast-enhancing, well-defined rim, and the presence of air bubbles.

Treatment

Abdominal abscesses should be drained; when an "active' source exists it should be dealt with, antibiotic treatment is of marginal importance.

Antibiotics

The truth is that no real evidence exists to prove that antimicrobial agents, which poorly-penetrate into an established abscess, are necessary at all – in addition to the complete evacuation of the pus. Think about the good old days – not many years ago, when pelvic abscesses were observed until reaching "maturity" and then drained through the rectum or the vagina; no antibiotics were used and the recovery was immediate and complete. The prevalent standard of care, however, although lacking evidence, maintains that when an abscess is strongly suspected or diagnosed then antibiotic therapy should be initiated. The latter should initially be empirically targeted against the usual expected polymicrobial spectrum of bacteria; when the causative bacteria are identified the coverage can be changed or reduced as indicated.

How Long to Administer Antibiotics?

Again there are no scientific data to formulate logical guidelines. Common-sense dictates that prolonged administration after the effective drainage is not necessary. Theoretically antibiotics may combat bacteremia during drainage and eradicate locally spilled microorganisms; but after the pus has been evacuated – leading to a clinical response – antibiotics should be discontinued. The presence of a drain is not an indication to continue with administration (chapter 32).

Conservative Treatment

Traditionally, multiple hepatic abscesses, as a consequence to portal pyemia, which are not amenable to drainage, are treated with antibiotics, with a variable response rate. There are those who claim that non-operative treatment, with prolonged administration of antibiotics, is also effective in children who develop abdominal abscesses following an appendectomy for acute appendicitis. The problem with such "successes" is that the

alleged "abscesses", which were imagined on US or CT, were never proven
as such. Instead, it probably represented sterile collections – the majority
requiring no therapy at all.

Drainage

Philosophy & timing

Presently the prevailing paradigm, when an abscess is suspected on a CT
or US, is to hit the patient with antibiotics and rush to drainage. In the
hysterical hurry "to treat", clinical lessons learned over centuries are often
ignored. Only a generation ago, a patient who spiked temperature after an
appendectomy was patiently but carefully observed without antibiotics
(which did not exist); usually the temperature – signifying residual local
inflammatory response syndrome (LIRS) (chapter 38) – subsided spontaneously. In the minority of patients "septic" fever persisted reflecting maturing
local suppuration. The later was eventually drained through the rectum when
assessed as "mature". Today, conversely, antibiotics are immediately given
to mask the clinical picture, and imaging techniques are instantly ordered
to diagnose "red herrings", which in turn promote unnecessary invasive
procedures. Remember: in a stable patient fever is a *symptom* of effective
host defenses – not an indication to be aggressively invasive (chapter 33).

Practical Approach

When an abscess is suspected a few dilemmas arise and should be dealt
with stepwise:

- *Is it an abscess or a sterile collection?* The aforementioned CT features
  may be helpful but the clinical scenario is as important – especially
  when *postoperative* abscesses are concerned. Abscesses rarely
  mature for drainage before a week has passed since the operation
  and three weeks after the operation the cause of "sepsis" is rarely
  within the abdomen. When in doubt image-guided diagnostic
  aspiration is indicated.

310
- *Percutaneous (PC) versus open surgical drainage?* During the 1980's multiple retrospective series suggested that the results of PC drainage are at least as good as that achieved by an operation. It was also said by some that, paradoxically, despite the attractiveness of a PC technique for abscess drainage in the most ill patients, a better chance for survival is achieved with surgical treatment, and that surgical treatment should not be avoided because the patient is considered to be too ill. Be that as it may, there is no clear evidence to attribute lesser mortality or morbidity to PC drainage versus surgical drainage. The former, however, represent a minimally-invasive procedure which can spare the patient the unpleasantness of another open abdominal operation.
- *The concept of a complex abscess is clinically useful* . Abscesses which are multiple, mutiloculated, associated with tissue necrosis, enteric communication or tumor – are defined as *complex* and poorly respond to PC drainage while most *simple* abscesses do. In gravely ill patients with *complex* abscesses, PC drainage may offer significant *temporizing* therapeutic benefits – allowing a definitive semi-elective laparotomy in better-stabilized patients.
- *It appears that PC drainage and surgical drainage techniques should not be considered competitive but rather complementary.* If an abscess is accessible by PC techniques, it is reasonable to consider a non-operative approach to the problem. You – the surgeon – should consider each abscess individually together with the radiologist, taking into the consideration the "pro & cons" presented in table 35–2.
- *Percutaneous aspiration only versus catheter drainage?* A single PC needle aspiration may successfully eradicate an abscess – especially when small and containing low-viscosity fluid. There is good evidence, however, that PC catheter drainage is more effective.
- *Size of PC catheters-drains?* Some claim advantage for large-bore trocar catheters for PC drainage but the evidence indicates however that size 7 French PC sump drains are as effective as size14 French.

- *Management of PC drains*: There is not much science here; these
  are small tubes and should be regularly flushed with saline to
  remain patent. The drain site should be regularly cleaned and
  observed: there are single case reports of necrotizing fasciitis of
  the abdominal wall around a PC drain site. *PC drains are removed*
  when clinical SIRS has resolved and the daily output (minus the
  saline injected) is below 25 ml. On the average, after PC drainage of
  a simple abdominal abscess the drain is removed after seven days.
- *Re-imaging*: A clinical improvement should be seen within 24 to
  72 hours following PC drainage. Persistent fever and leukocytosis
  at the fourth day after PC drainage correlates with a management
  failure. Non-responders should be re-imagined with a CT-combined
  with water-soluble contrast injected through the drain. Depending
  on the finding a decision should be taken by you – the surgeon – in
  consultation with the radiologist, as to the next appropriate course
  of action – a re-PC drain or an operation. Persistence of high output
  drainage in a patient who is clinically well can be better investigated
  with a tube sinogram to delineate the size of the residual abscess
  cavity. Abscess cavities which do not collapse commonly recur.

Failure of PC Drainage: When to "Switch Over" to Surgical Drainage?

Patients who deteriorate after the first attempt at PC drainage should be operated upon promptly; further procrastination may be disastrous.

In stable non-responders to the initial PC drainage a second attempt may be appropriate, according to the considerations mentioned in - table 35.2. Inability to successfully affect the second PC drainage, or its clinical failure, mandates an open procedure.

Table 35.2. Intra-abdominal abscesses: percutaneous (PC) versus open surgical drainage. Considerations in selecting the approach.

	PC drainage	Open drainage
Surgically accessibility	"Hostile" abdomen	Accessible
PC accessibility	Yes	No
Source controlled	Yes	No
Location	Visceral	interloop
Number abscesses	Single	Multiple
Loculated	No	Yes
Communication with bowel	No	Yes
Associated necrosis	No	Yes
Associated malignancy	No	Yes
Contents	Thin	Thick debris
Invasive radiologist	Available	Not available
Severity off illness	"Stable"	Critically ill
Failed PC drainage	No	Yes

Surgical Management
of Intra-abdominal Abscesses

About a third of intra-abdominal abscesses are not suitable to PC drainage and require an open operation. A few practical dilemmas exist:

- *Exploratory laparotomy vs. "direct" surgical approach*: A "blind" exploratory laparotomy to search for abscesses – "somewhere", so common less than 20 years ago is currently very rarely necessary. A *"direct"* approach is obviously more "benign", sparing the previously uninvolved peritoneal spaces and avoiding bowel injury and wound complications. It is almost always possible in spontaneous abscesses, which are so well defined on CT. But those are also the kind of abscesses, which usually respond to PC drainage. Although postoperative abscesses are today anatomically well localized on

Table 35.3. Exploratory laparotomy vs. "direct" open drainage of abdominal abscesses.   313

	Exploratory laparotomy	"Direct" open drainage
Abscess accurately localized on CT	No	Yes
Early postoperative phase	Yes	No
Late postoperative phase	No	Yes
Single abscess	No	Yes
Multiple abscesses	Yes	No
Lesser sac abscess	Yes	No
Interloop abscess	Yes	No
Source of infection uncontrolled	Yes	No
Subphrenic/subhepatic	No	Yes
Gutter abscess	No	Yes
Pelvic	No	Yes

CT, those which fail PC drainage are usually "complex", thus often not amenable to a "direct" approach (e.g. interloop abscess) or requiring in addition the control of the intestinal source. Criteria for making the choice of the approach are summarized in table 35.3.

- *Direct approach: extra-peritoneal versus trans-peritoneal?* There are no significant differences in overall mortality and morbidly between the two approaches; the trans-peritoneal route is, however, associated with a higher incidence of injury to the bowel. It logical to suggest that the extra-peritoneal approach should be utilized whenever anatomically possible. *Subphrenic* and *subhepatic* abscesses can be approached extra-peritoneally through a subcostal incision or – if posterior-thorough the *bed of the 12th rib*. Old timers are still familiar with these techniques which are currently rarely utilized – being replaced by PC drainage. *Peri-colic, appendicular* (chapter 22) and all sorts of *retroperitoneal* abscesses are best approached through a *loin incision*. Also late-appearing *pancreatic* abscesses

314

(chapter 14) can be drained extra-peritoneally-from the flank-occasionally needing a bilateral approach. *Pelvic* abscesses are best drained *through the rectum or vagina.*

- *Drains?* Classically, at the end of the open procedure a drain has been placed within the abscess cavity – brought to the skin *away* from the main incision. The type, size and number of drains used depended more on local traditions and preferences than on science. Similarly, the postoperative management of drains involved cumbersome rituals with the drains sequentially shortened, based on serial contrast sinogram – to ascertain the gradual collapse of the cavities and drain-tracts. House surgeons and nurses forever changed dressings and irrigated the drains – again according to the locally prevailing ritual. Our experience is that this scenario should belong to history. With adequate surgical drainage, when the source of infection has been controlled, when the abscess cavity is "filled" with omentum or adjacent structures, and prophylactic peri-operative antibiotics are administered – no drains are necessary. Trust the peritoneal cavity to deal with the residual bacteria better in the absence of a foreign-body – a drain. We do not remember when was the last time we had to "shorten" a drain or to obtain a drain-sinogram. Oh, the sweet memories of youth.

Summary

Tailor your approach to the anatomy of the abscess, the physiology of the patient, and the local facilities available to you. Do not procrastinate, do not forget to deal with the source, do not over rely on antibiotics, and get rid off the pus. Sepsis – the host generated systemic inflammatory response to the abscess may persist, and progress to organ failure, even after the abscess has been adequately managed (chapter 38). Try not to be too late.

36 Abdominal Wall Dehiscence

*The gut bursts out either because you did not close the tummy properly
or it has no place inside...*

When rounding on your patient, who five days ago had a laparotomy for
intestinal obstruction, you find his wound dressings soaked in some
clear-pinkish fluid. "Change the dressings more frequently" you mutter
to the intern. A day later, during lunch, you are paged by the head nurse
on the floor: "Doctor, Mr. Hirsch's intestines are spread all around his
bed. Please come and help...!" How embarrassing.

Definitions

Abdominal dehiscence is either complete or partial, the latter being
much more common.

- *Partial* (covert, latent) dehiscence is a separation of the fascial
  edges of the wound without evisceration or full exposure of the
  underlying viscera. It presents usually a few days after the operation
  with some sero-sanguinous peritoneal fluid seeping through the
  wound. When the skin edges are separated or if, as commonly
  occurs, wound infection is present, you may see the exposed fascia,
  loose fascial sutures, and occasionally a fibrin-covered loop of
  intestine
- *Complete* dehiscence is full a separation of the fascia and skin.
  Loops of intestine – if not glued in place by adhesions – commonly
  eviscerate "all over the place".

316   Etiology

Multiple local, mechanical and systemic factors contribute to abdominal wound dehiscence: wound infection, pulmonary disease, hemodynamic instability, ostomies in the wound, age >65, hypoalbuminemia, systemic infection, obesity, uremia, TPN, malignancy, ascites, corticosteroid use and hypertension. These are factors, which cause poor tissue healing and/or an increased intra-abdominal pressure. A few of these factors are present in any patient who suffers a dehiscence. Dehiscence, be it complete or partial, is associated with a significant mortality rate. The prevailing perception is that the M & M associated with dehiscence is caused by the underlying local and systemic factors leading to the dehiscence, the latter representing only a marker for the former, rather than the cause of death. However, the way dehiscence is managed has also impact on the outcome, as you'll see below.

How To Prevent Dehiscence?

In essence you can prevent dehiscence by:
- Choosing a "correct" incision (chapter 8)
- "Correctly" closing the abdomen (chapter 29)
- Not closing abdomens which should be left open (chapters 28 & 37)

Generally, it appears that vertical incisions – especially the midline – are associated with a greater incidence of dehiscence than transverse incisions. In mechanical terms, *three main causes for dehiscence exist: the suture breaks, the knot slips, or the tissue breaks* (i.e. the suture cuts through the tissues). The last mentioned is the dominant one. Please re-read chapter 29 to ingrain in your brain how dehiscence can be prevented by "correct" abdominal closure. And, remember, that abdomens which are very likely to burst out could be left open as discussed elsewhere in this book (chapters 28 & 37).

Treatment

"Leading" surgical texts advocate an immediate surgical 'closure" of the dehiscence. For example, Schwartz's textbook recommends that "If the patient can tolerate the procedure, a secondary operative procedure is indicated". What kind of a patient "cannot tolerate the procedure" is not stated. The guidelines published by the American College of Surgeons state that if "dehiscence is significant an immediate operative re-closure is preferred ". A text devoted to complications in surgery suggests that "when a dressing is found soaked in salmon-pink fluid...a fascial defect or a loop of bowel palpated just below the skin...binder must be applied and the patient sent promptly to the operating room". In addition, "failure to repair dehiscence results in evisceration in most cases...re-closure, in contrast is strikingly successful". Another recent text on re-operative general surgery emphasizes that "abdominal wound dehiscence is clearly a surgical emergency" requiring fascial re-closure.

Managed according to the above recommendations patients are taken to the operating room where their abdomen are re-sutured with "retention sutures" (see chapter 29). So why is the mortality so high? Many still think that "most deaths associated with dehiscence today are the result of ongoing primary disease rather than being a direct result of this complication". There is a large body of data, however, to suggest that such hypothesis is not true. Instead, it appears that the "recommended" treatment of the dehiscence-re-closure-plays a significant role in the associated M & M.

We believe that that forcing the distended intestines back into a cavity of limited size may kill the patient. The *fatal factor* leading to the high mortality rate associated with abdominal wound dehiscence is not the dehiscence itself but the emergency procedure to correct it, which produces intra-abdominal hypertension, which in turn adversely affected cardiovascular, respiratory, renal and intestinal function, leading to multi-organ dysfunction and eventually death (chapter 28).

318   Recommended Approach to Dehiscence

Instead of routinely "pushing back" the bulging viscera into the limited space of the peritoneal cavity, be selective – using the following rational:

- *Complete dehiscence mandates* an operation to reduce the eviscerated abdominal contents. You cannot leave the intestine hanging outside the bed. You may attempt a re-closure of the fascia when a faulty closure technique or a broken suture is the cause of the dehiscence and local circumstances permit. If this is the case, approximate the facial edges towards each other, while measuring intra-abdominal pressure through the urinary catheter (chapter 28). A pressure higher than 25 cm' water would deter us from primary closure. Instead, we would choose to leave the abdomen temporary open, using one of the TACD methods described in chapter 37. We would avoid re-closure also when the abdominal wall is "frail" or if the cause of the evisceration – persistent intra-abdominal infection-is still present. *What is the use of re-suturing the abdomen if the factors causing its evisceration in the first place are still present?*

- *Partial dehiscence may be managed conservatively.* Many surgeons feel compelled to take the patient to the operating room and re-suture the fascia. But what's the rush? In our experience this is not only unnecessary but may even complicate matters. The natural course of a partially dehisced wound is to heal by granulation and scarring with or without the formation of an incisional hernia. Re-suturing such a friable wound in a compromised patient entails the additive risks of anesthesia and abdominal re-entry while not preventing the eventual hernia. The latter, if symptomatic, can be repaired electively in a later stage. If the bowel were partially exposed we would approximate the skin to cover it. Otherwise, the wound is managed as any open wound (chapter 40) until healing.

Summary

In most instances dehiscence is more a *symptom rather than a disease.*
Operate for complete dehiscence with evisceration; re-suture fascia or
use TACD selectively. Most cases of partial dehiscence are best treated
conservatively.

37 Re-laparotomies and Laparostomy for Infection

A negative re-laparotomy is better than a positive autopsy but is not, nevertheless, a benign procedure.

Remember chapter 10 where we discussed the principles of management of *intra-abdominal infection (IAI)*? We told you that in some patients, to improve survival, the performance of *source* and *damage* control must be repeated: certain patients need a *re-laparotomy*. In this chapter we'll discuss re-laparotomies in greater detail. Leaving the abdomen-open or *laparostomy* is a common corollary to re-laparotomies; hence, it is discussed here as well. Before we continue you should be re-introduced to some definitions.

"On-Demand" Versus "Planned" Re-laparotomy

There are two types of re-laparotomies:
- *"On-demand"*: when, in the aftermath of an initial laparotomy, evidence of an intra-abdominal complication forces the surgeon to re-operate.
- *"Planned"* (or "electively-staged"): when, at the initial laparotomy, the surgeon takes the decision to re-operate within 1-3 days, irrespective of his or her patient's immediate postoperative course.

Both these types of re-laparotomies have a place in the postoperative management of the patient following a laparotomy, but they apply in different clinical contexts.

322   ### *Re-laparotomy "on Demand"*

The unexpected development of IAI after an initial-"index" laparotomy constitutes the indication for such a re-look. The two postoperative complications requiring a re-look are generalised *peritonitis* and *intra-abdominal abscess*. A post-operative suture-line or anastomotic dehiscence may manifest itself either as an external fistula, with no peritoneal contamination, or as a peritonitis – be it generalised or localised (i.e. abscesses). Leaks take place typically between the 5th and 8th postoperative day, but may occur earlier or later (see also chapters 35 and 39).

Peritonitis complicating a laparotomy is termed *"postoperative peritonitis"*. This is one of the most lethal types of peritonitis – killing between one-third to half of the patients – for the following two reasons:

- Its diagnosis is usually delayed because the abdominal signs (tenderness, distension...) are initially masked by the expected similar signs of the postoperative abdomen.
- It occurs in the postoperative phase, when the patient is catabolic, already "inflamed" by SIRS and immunodepressed by CARS (chapter 38).

There are several possible clinical presentations developing within days of a laparotomy:

- *Generalised peritonitis.* The abdominal findings are out of proportion to the "normal" postoperative state (severe abdominal pain and tenderness, massive or prolonged ileus); there may be associated systemic repercussions (fever, leukocytosis) that are uncharacteristic of the expected postoperative recovery. Sometimes, the diagnosis is made easier by additional presence of an entero-cutaneous fistula (chapter 39), deep wound infection (chapter 40) or abdominal wall dehiscence (chapter 37).
- *Organ dysfunction. (Renal failure or "atelectasis"/"pneumonia" – in fact an incipient ARDS).* Not infrequently, the unsuspecting surgeon seeks expert advice from medical colleagues (nephrologist, chest

physician, infection disease specialist or intensivist). Of course, renal failure or pneumonia may well occur in a postoperative patient for a variety of reasons that are unrelated to an intra-abdominal complication. But similarly, an IAI may also present initially as a single system dysfunction and progress, in time, to multiple organ failure. It is essential, firstly, to be aware of the relationship between IAI and organ dysfunction (chapter 38) and, secondly, to be humble enough to consider the possibility of such a complication in one's patient (chapter 33). The diagnosis is established by careful clinical evaluation of the abdomen, supplemented if necessary with computed tomography (CT).

- *The intensive care setting.* The possibility of IAI is raised because of the need for prolonged ventilation or aggravation of the multiple organ dysfunction in a critically ill postoperative patient after massive trauma or major abdominal surgery. Intensivists are usually quick to point to the abdomen as the culprit and eager to spur the surgeon to re-explore. In a ventilated, paralysed patient, the abdomen cannot be evaluated clinically. There is therefore a real dilemma in differentiating between the presence of an abdominal focus of infection and the systemic inflammatory response syndrome (SIRS) without infection (chapter 38). Abdominal CT is claimed by radiologists to be very useful but unfortunately is not. After any laparotomy, tissue planes are distorted and potential spaces may contain fluid; even the best radiologist cannot tell you whether the fluid is blood, serous, leaking bowel contents or pus. In addition, transporting a critically ill patient on maximal organ support to the CT suit is not an innocuous procedure. Diagnostic peritoneal lavage – evaluating the lavage fluid for its macroscopic characteristics (feces, pus, bile, and blood) smell, and bacteria (Gram stain and culture) is occasionally helpful and can be done at the bedside. The decision to re-operate, however, can be extremely difficult to make and requires good co-operation between surgeons, intensivists (who hopefully are also surgeons) and radiologists.
- Intra-abdominal abscess (see chapter 35).

324   *"Planned" ("Electively Staged") Re-laparotomy*

The decision to re-explore the abdomen (usually within 24-72 hours) is made at the time of the initial laparotomy and is part of the management plan. Historically, mesenteric ischemia is probably the first instance when a planned re-look laparotomy was advocated (chapter 19). Having resected ischemic bowel and performed an anastomosis in the setting of precarious vascularity, the surgeon decides to re-look the abdomen in order to check the viability of the anastomosis. In the context of intra-abdominal infection, the justification for a re-look is to anticipate the re-formation of infected collections and to prevent the persistence or development of SIRS and multiple organ failure. The indications for a planned re-laparotomy are:

- *Severe diffuse peritonitis.* For example massive or long-standing fecal peritonitis or postoperative suture line dehiscence ("post-operative peritonitis"). The indication for the re-operation is based on the empirical knowledge that, in this setting, a once-for-all operation is commonly unsuccessful: purulent collections re-form and may eventually be responsible for multiple organ failure.
- *Whenever the initial pathological entity-source – cannot be controlled definitively at the first laparotomy.* A good example is the infected retroperitoneal tissue associated with infected pancreatic necrosis (chapter 14). It often is an evolving pathological process with on-going formation of infected slough, which requires repeated debridement.

The Conduct of a Re-laparotomy

The key advice for the surgeon who plans to return into a recently operated upon abdomen is to *be gentle*! The peritoneal surfaces are edematous, friable and vascular; so is the bowel. Re-operative abdominal surgery is

one of the few real scenarios where the dictum "first do not harm" is
crucial. Do not produce holes in bowel, do not cause bleeding – such
mishaps could kill your already compromised patient.

Another important tip: *know your way around*. Ideally, the surgeon
who has performed the original-"index" procedure should be the one to
re-operate or at least be among the re-operating team. Think about the
infected postoperative abdomen as a thick jungle: a previous journey
through it renders a re-visit easier. You will remember, for example, that
the colon was "sticking" to the lower end of the incision; your partner,
on the other hand, who did not visit this abdomen before, will immediately enter the lumen of the colon – with horrendous consequences.

The abdominal re-look itself aims at draining all infected collections
and controlling, if necessary, persistent sources of contamination. How
thorough the exploration depends on the individual case. Sometimes
there are several inter-loop abscesses that need to be drained and the
whole bowel must be carefully unravelled; in other cases, particularly in
instances of frozen abdomen, it is sufficient to explore the spaces around
the matted bowel (subphrenic spaces, paracolic gutters, pelvis). The
decision about the extent of exploration is crucial because the more
widespread it is, the more danger it poses to adjacent structures. And, as
you were told here again and again – the more you do – the more local
and systemic inflammation you create. *The "extent" of exploration then
depends on whether your operation is "directed" or "non-directed" and on
its timing.*

"Directed" Versus "Non-directed" Re-look

"Directed" re-operation means that you know exactly where you want to
go and what for. The CT showed a right subhepatic collection, with the
rest of the abdomen appearing "clean". You can "go" directly into where
the action is – sparing the rest of the abdomen the potentially damaging
effects of your hands and instruments. Conversely, a "non-directed" re-

look is a "blind" re-exploration when you are not sure where the "problem" exactly lies; for example, CT showed free fluid everywhere – here you are forced to search "all around".

Timing of Re-Look

When you re-explore the abdomen 24–72 hours after the initial operation the adhesions between the viscera and peritoneal surfaces are easily separable; you can enter any space with atraumatic dissection. At this stage, "total" abdominal exploration is readily accomplishable. As time passes by, the intra-abdominal structures are progressively cemented to each other with, dense, vascular, immature adhesions – which are troublesome to divide. Clearly, abdominal re-entry within 7 days to 4 weeks of the "index" operation may be hazardous – until the eventual maturation of the adhesions which takes many weeks to occur.

Consequently, during an "early" re-look operation you may separate all loops of bowels – getting rid of intra-loop collections. At "late" re-operations, however, you will find a *central mass of matted small bowel*. Leave it alone! Dissection of the individual loops at this stage is dangerous and non-productive, as significant collections are to be found at the periphery: *above* – under the diaphragms, under the liver; *below* – in the pelvis and on the *sides* – in the gutters.

During re-exploration sharp dissection is rarely needed. Your fingers are the best exploratory instruments – dissecting into the spaces. *Remember*; where tissue plans are normal – not readily admitting your dissecting, pinching fingers – nothing is to be found. So follow your fingers, which lead you into where the pus lies.

The Leaking Intestine

Dehisced suture lines and anastomoses must be de-functioned, ideally by the fashioning of appropriate stomas or, if this is not possible, by tube drainage.

Re-suturing leaking bowel in an infected peritoneal cavity is doomed to   327
failure and carries a high mortality. Much more on this issue see in chapter 39.

Drains

The use of intraperitoneal drains is controversial in this setting. It is
certainly obviated if the decision is taken to re-explore in a few days later.
The placement of a drain at the final laparotomy may be considered; the
advantages need to be weighed against the risk of damage to viscera that
are extremely friable as a result of recent re-explorations (chapter 33).

When to Stop?

As in most vital aspects in life, too much of anything is hurtful: too many
"planned re-laparotomies" are harmful. When to stop? In a management
program of planned re-looks the decision to discontinue the re-explorations
must be based on the finding of a macroscopically clean peritoneal cavity
and evidence that sources of contamination have been controlled definitively.
Whether the source is controlled or not is obvious but estimation whether
the peritoneal cavity is "clean" or not requires experience and judgement.

When peritonitis persists despite adequate source control and repeated re-operations – think about *tertiary peritonitis* (chapter 38).

Laparostomy

The open management of the infected abdomen (laparostomy) was instituted in the belief that the peritoneal cavity could be treated like an abscess
cavity. It soon became clear, however, that there was still a need for thorough
abdominal re-explorations in search for deep pockets of infected collections. Laparostomy has now become a corollary to the policy of repeated
laparotomies; indeed, if the abdomen is to be re-looked 48 hours later, why

328   close it at all? The potential advantages of the technique are substantial. Necrosis of the macerated abdominal midline closed forcefully and repeatedly in the presence of an edematous and distended bowel is avoided; a better diaphragmatic excursion may be expected; the abdominal compartment syndrome with its renal, respiratory and hemodynamic repercussions is prevented (chapter 28). Complications do occur however: spontaneous enteric fistulas, fluid losses, hypothermia and risk of evisceration. The use of *temporary abdominal cover devise* (*TACD*) of the abdominal defect by a synthetic mesh, or other means, has minimised these complications. Nevertheless, practical problems associated with the implementation of this technique persist, and there is always a need for subsequent reconstruction of the abdominal wall.

Laparostomy is indicated when a satisfactory abdominal closure is impossible or may be used in selected cases; the build of the patient, the volume of infected exudate, the degree of ileus and intestinal parietal edema, the status of the wound edges and the number of anticipated re-operations should all be taken into consideration. *For practical purposes think that laparostomy may be indicated either when the abdomen cannot be closed or should not be closed.*

Abdomen Which Cannot Be Closed

- After major loss of abdominal-wall tissue following trauma or debridement for necrotizing fasciitis.
- Extreme visceral or retroperitoneal swelling and bulging after major trauma, resuscitation, or major surgery (e.g. rupture AAA).
- Poor condition of fascia after multiple laparotomies.

Abdomen Which Should Not Be Closed

- Plan to re-operate within a day or two – why lock the gate through which you are to re-enter very soon?

- Closure possible only under extreme tension – compromising the   329
  fascia and raising intra-abdominal pressure.

Technical Consideration of Laparostomy

You decided not to close the abdomen; how should you manage it? The
option of simply covering the exposed viscera with moist gauze packs has
been practised for generations but is inadvisable: the intestine – if not
matted – can eviscerate; it is messy – requiring intensive work to keep the
patient and his bed clean and dry. But above all, it has an established risk
of creating spontaneous "exposed" intestinal fistulas (chapter 39). The
exposed bowel, when dilated and friable, tends to "pop" when repeatedly
injured by caring nurses and interns. *TACD* is therefore highly recommended; but which TACD?

Your local guru-mentor has probably his own preferred method of
TACD, be it a "Bogota bag" made off a large IV fluid bag, a ready to use
transparent "bowel bag", a synthetic mesh (absorbable or non-absorbable),
or a Velcro-type sheath. We even know a guy in South America who uses
discarded nylon hose for this purpose. In fact, what you chose to use probably
does not matter but there are a few practical points worth remembering:

- Whichever TACD you use, try to place it over the omentum – if available.
- Suture the TACD to the fascial edges. Just placing it "on top" will result
  in huge abdominal – wall defects because the midline – wound fascial
  edges tend to retract laterally (note that this is the reason why the abdominal defect resulting from a *transverse* laparostomy is smaller).
  The larger the defect the more problematic its eventual reconstruction.
- Using a permeable TACD (i.e. mesh) as opposed to a non-perme-
  able (e.g. Bogota bag) has the advantage of allowing the egress of
  infected intra-peritoneal fluids.
- Try to adjust the tension of TACD to the IAP (chapter 28).
- If you plan another re-operation the type of TACD you use is of
  little importance: you can always replace the TACD at the end of the

next laparotomy. The selection of TACD when no more re-opera-tion are deemed necessary is crucial; we recommend an *absorbable synthetic mesh* as discussed below.

- Abdominal re-entry through the TACD is simple: divide the TACD at its centre; with your finger gently separate the omentum and viscera away from the overlying TACD. At the end of the procedure re-suture the TACD devise with a running suture. Zippers can be used instead: an attractive gimmick to nurses and interns.

Our own TACD of choice is the "sandwich technique": an absorbable permeable synthetic mesh is sutured to the fascial edges. Two tubes (sump drains) are placed at the sides of the abdominal defect – over the mesh, connected to suction – to collect the abdominal effluents. Sheaths of stoma-adhesive are placed on the healthy skin surrounding the defect; a large adhesive transparent sheath ("Steridrape" or "Opsite") is placed "on top" to cover the entire abdomen. Hence, the viscera are protected, the laparostomy's output measurable, the patient is clean and dry with demands on nursing minimised (figure 37.1).

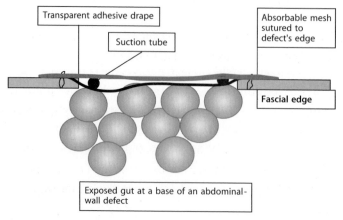

Figure 37.1. The "sandwich technique" in the management of laparostomy.

Terminating the Laparostomy

How to treat the ensuing abdominal-wall defect when the reason to
initiate laparostomy exists no more?
- If non-absorbable material has been used as a TACD, it must be
  removed. Leaving pieces of Marlex mesh in the depth of such a
  defect will results in a chronic mess of infected sinuses and even
  intestinal fistulas.
- Occasionally, when the defect is small it may be possible to close it
  completely. If the healthy surrounding skin comes nicely together
  forget about fascia and close the skin above the defect. Laterally
  placed "relaxation incision" occasionally help to bring the midline
  together. The sure to develop hernia is of minor importance at this
  stage. In most patients recovering from multiple re-laparotomies
  and laparostomy the defect is too large, however, to allow primary
  closure of the fascia or skin. Hence, the safest option is to let the
  defect to granulate under and over the absorbable mesh. In a week
  or two after the last laparotomy, when healthy layer of granulation
  tissue has covered the omentum and viscera and the patient's recovery is well under way, split-skin graft is easily applied onto the
  granulation tissue in the defect's bed. The resulting ventral hernia
  is usually wide-necked and well tolerated except for its cosmetic
  appearance. It can be repaired at a later stage.
- Now you understand why the use of an absorbable synthetic mesh
  (e.g. Vicryl or Dexon) as a "final" TACD is advantageous. It can be
  left in situ to rapidly disintegrate within the granulating abdominal
  defect – to be skin grafted.
- Whatever you do with the abdominal-wall defect remember that
  your patient has just recovered from the immense stress of peritonitis and multiple operations: he cannot take much more at this
  stage.

332   Antibiotics

As mentioned in chapter 32, in patients with severe intra-abdominal infection who "deserve" re-operations and/or laparostomy for additional source and damage control, prolonged courses of postoperative antibiotics are justified. Antibiotics should be continued as long as the source, and residual infection, is "active". Recent evidence suggests that in this sub-group of patients anti-fungal prophylaxis with fluconazole may decrease the incidence of intra-abdominal superinfection with *Candida* species.

Conclusions

Relaparotomies and *laparostomy* are therapeutic measures that are indicated in a minority of patients. They represent, for the time being, the heaviest weaponry in the surgeon's mechanical armamentarium for the treatment of severe intra-abdominal infection and other post-laparotomy abdominal catastrophes. It is well to remind us that unnecessary re-laparotomies carry significant morbidity. An aggressive but selective policy of directed "on-demand" re-looks, supplemented by laparostomy, if necessary, is probably superior to a "blind" execution of planned re-laparotomies. *Source and damage control-above all!*

38 LIRS, SIRS, Sepsis, MODS and Tertiary Peritonitis

The larger the operation – the greater is the trauma
The greater is the trauma – the stronger is the SIRS
The stronger is the SIRS – the sicker is the patient
The sicker is the patient – the higher is his M & M

Already in the first paragraph of this book we alluded to your patient as being *locally and systemically inflamed* – by his surgical disease, your treatment, and the complications of both. Almost at each subsequent chapter you were reminded that the magnitude of the inflammation correlates with that of the disease process and the operation. You were told that the more inflammation there is – or that you create – the more is your patient likely to develop organ dysfunction or failure and to die. In this chapter, we'll concentrate on the inflammation – be it local or systemic – and its consequences. The biological events involved are immense and chaotic but let us maintain a simplistic attitude – you did not buy this book to read about cytokines, right?

Background

Matters were much simpler for us – clinical surgeons – only a few years ago. Post operative or post-traumatic fever, raised white cell count, sliding-down organ-system function, with or without "shock", meant for us only one thing – "sepsis". And "sepsis" meant "infection", usually bacterial in nature, necessitating antibiotic therapy. So we administered the "strongest", ever-changing, antimicrobial agents available on the market, we looked for pus – draining it whenever present, and we prayed for the "infection" to subside. Some of our patients, however, continued to deteriorate, dying

334   slowly from respiratory and/or renal failure. We buried them, blaming
the death on an "intractable sepsis", which in our minds always signified
an infection – "somewhere" in their blood, abdomen, urine or lungs.
Look around you – isn't this the way many of your senior colleagues,
mentors or teachers still think and practice?

Then, in the early 1980's, when our supportive care and re-operative
efforts became more aggressive – resulting in prolonged survival, we begun
to note that many of our patients were dying a "septic" death in the absence
of "infection"; we did not understand why. Towards the second half of the
1980's a rapidly developing field of molecular biology produced a huge
amount of data to explain that a lot of what we see in clinical practice is
not "sepsis" or "infection" but *inflammation* – which in turn is fueled by
pro-inflammatory mediators-*cytokines*. This has totally changed the way
we begun to look at the surgical patient. We see him being *inflamed* by
the disease, the operative trauma as well as by the postoperative complications and their therapies. But before we go further, we need to clarify a
few issues in terminology.

Terminology

Take a knife and cut yourself in a finger: sooner or later your finger will
manifest the usual signs of inflammation – redness, swelling, warmth
and pain – produced by locally produced inflammatory mediators. This
is *LIRS – local inflammatory response syndrome*.

Now take a patient who suffered multiple, and deeper, knife wounds
to the soft tissues: in addition to the local inflammation he'll experience
signs of systemic inflammation: fever, tachycardia and even elevation of
his white cell count. This is *SIRS – or systemic inflammatory response
syndrome*. SIRS occurs when the locally pro-inflammatory mediators of
LIRS-spill over to the systemic circulation – affecting the entire organism.
In surgical practice most instances of SIRS are secondary to LIRS – such

as acute pancreatitis, retroperitoneal hemorrhage or acute cholecystitis.   335
*Note that the pro-inflammatory cascades leading to SIRS are initially, at
least, well compartmentalized locally, with the SIRS representing only the
tip of the iceberg.*

LIRS and SIRS are caused by sterile-non infective causes (e.g. tissue trauma, necrosis, burn) as well as infective causes (e.g. acute appendicitis). Clinical manifestation are however indistinguishable.

Infection – is a microbiological phenomenon – characterized by
the invasion of normally sterile tissue by microorganisms. The host's local response to the infection is LIRS – the systemic is SIRS. And here we
arrive at the term *sepsis*:

Sepsis is currently defined as the systemic response to *infection*
consisting of *SIRS* with microbiological evidence of infection. (*Sepsis=in-
flammation (SIRS) + infection*). In other words, *SIRS* and *sepsis* represent
an identical host-determined response, the former in culture negative
patients and the latter when infection is documented. Both manifest
a continuum of clinical and pathophysiologic severity.

According to current consensus SIRS may be diagnosed in any
patient who manifests two or more of the following: temperature 38°C
(100.4°F), heart rate >90/min, respiratory rate >20/min, white cell
count>12,000 cells/mm^3. With such a low inclusion threshold, it appears
that most of your emergency abdominal postoperative patients, and all
your SICU cases, experience a degree SIRS. (In fact, there was someone
who said that even engaging in vigorous sex produces clinical SIRS).

The obnoxious stimuli, which incite *pro-inflammatory* mediators,
thus LIRS and SIRS – induce in parallel potent anti-inflammatory
mediators, to produce what the late Roger Bone (the "father" of SIRS)
termed *CARS – compensatory anti-inflammatory syndrome*. CARS manifests clinically as immunodepression and an increased susceptibility to
infection, so typical in the aftermath of major surgery and trauma.
Conceptually, the balance between SIRS and CARS determines outcome:
when CARS equalizes SIRS – homeostasis results; when SIRS is unop-

336   posed – organ dysfunction develops; when CARS is the winner – primary or secondary infections may take their toll.

As with many other essential things in life, too much may be harmful and too little may be not satisfactory. The same probably is true for the inflammatory and anti-inflammatory responses, which in a certain phase and magnitude are beneficial but when out of control are harmful. Understand, however, that these events are extremely complex, chaotic, non-linear and unpredictable: some severely traumatized patients do not progress from SIRS to organ failure and some do. Your grand mother may be right – genes play a role in everything.

From SIRS – to Multi-Organ Dysfunction Syndrome (MODS)

The same pro-inflammatory mediators which locally posses salutary actions, when over-produced and systemically spread, eventually damage the microcirculation – resulting in progressive damage to vital organs. Your SIRS patient swells; he gains weight, his lungs become wet, the gastric mucosa bleeds, liver enzymes become elevated, renal dysfunction appears, and so forth. The patients become autointoxicated with his own inflammatory mediators. The more severe is the damage to the organs, the more organs are involved and for a longer duration – the less likely is your patient to recover. When more than three organs fail the prognosis is grim; when the fourth organ joins in – all efforts become futile.

The Second Hit Phenomena

Imagine a boxer in a ring. Having just received a major blow he lifts himself up, back on his feet; almost erect he receives a second hit which is softer than the first one, but enough to send the boxer back onto the floor – a knock out. Similarly, your SIRS patient is susceptible to a second

hit: his inflammatory response being switched on by the primary hit is
easily amplified by additional, albeit relatively minor hits. Think about
your patient as about an aging boxer: the abdominal emergency plus
your operation represent the first hit – from now on any additional
procedure or a complication constitute a potential second hit, which
increases the magnitude of the inflammation.

Treatment of SIRS and MODS

The search for the magic bullet to arrest the cascades of LIRS, SIRS and
to modulate CARS continues; but meanwhile is there anything we can do
for these patients?

- First, we need to use terms accurately, distinguishing between local
  inflammation and infection, between SIRS and systemic sepsis. We
  must understand that LIRS and SIRS do not always mean infection
  and thus may not be an indication to administer antibiotics (chapter 10 & 32).
- Second, we must restore and maintain perfusion of end organs to
  prevent an on-going and additional ischemic injury – which contributes to the inflammation (chapter 5).
- Third, we must avoid adding fuel to the inflammatory fire, apprecia-
  ting that what we do, and how extensive we do things does matters.
  "Greater" operations and rough handling of tissues means more inflammation – more LIRS and SIRS. Unnecessary and poorly timed re-
  interventions may produce a "second hit" in a previously primed host.
- Fourth, we should promptly deal with ongoing infective (e.g., an
  abscess) and non-infective (e.g. necrotic tissue) sources of LIRS
  and SIRS.
- Fifth, we should attempt to preserve the integrity of the mucosal
  layer of the gut (through early feeding) in order to prevent translocation of bacteria and endotoxin – which may contribute to SIRS,
  sepsis and MODS (chapter 31).

- Sixth, we should minimize iatrogenic contributors to LIRS and SIRS: the patient must not be continuously injured and crucified in bed with indiscriminate insertion of catheters, tubes and pipes. Blood products may be harmful and should be used only as necessary (chapter 33). Antibiotics represent a double-edged sword and may in fact increase SIRS by various mechanisms.

It is impossible to prove that each of the above measures decreases SIRS and MODS; but proper management as a whole is the mainstay of prevention of this so-called "horror autotoxicus".

Tertiary Peritonitis

In chapter 10 you were introduced with the concepts of peritoneal contamination and infection and the terms *primary and secondary peritonitis*. The last chapter you read – chapter 37 – stated: "When peritonitis persists despite adequate source control and repeated re-operations – think about tertiary peritonitis". What's that?

The aggressive supportive and operative measures, discussed in the previous chapter – allow the initial salvage of patients who previously would have succumbed early to uncontrolled secondary peritonitis. This success however created a new subgroup of patients. Let us take one as an example:

> A 75 years old male underwent an emergency subtotal colectomy with an ileorectal anastomosis for an obstructing carcinoma of the sigmoid colon (chapter 21). Six days later he was rushed for a re-laparotomy because of diffuse peritonitis and a documented free anastomotic leak. At operation his abdomen was found to be full with bowel contents; it was cleansed and the anastomosis was dismantled; the rectum was closed as a Hartmann's pouch and the ileum exteriorized as an end ileostomy. The abdomen was left open as a 'laparostomy' During a planned relaparotomy 48 hour later residual collections of 'thin' pus were evacuated. The patient continued to

be 'septic' and developed MODS. CT of the abdomen showed fluid in the pelvis and gutters; diagnostic aspiration revealed the presence of fungi. An anti-fungal agent was added to the wide spectrum antibiotics the patient was already receiving. He continued to deteriorate; a re-laparotomy disclosed a few hundred ml of murky peritoneal fluid – which grew *candida* and *Stap. Epidermidis*. The antibiotics regimen was changed. MODS worsened leading to the patient's demise 5 weeks after the first operation. The hospital bill was $ 250,000.

You have seen similar patients, eh? Probably one of them is now fading away in your ICU. The term *tertiary peritonitis* was coined to describe this situation, which develops late in the postoperative phase, manifests clinically as SIRS with MODS, and is associated with a peculiar peritoneal microbiology consisting of yeasts, and other commensulas. The low virulence of these organisms represents probably a marker of tertiary peritonitis and not its cause. This also reflects the global immunodepression of the affected patient, allowing superinfection of the re-explored abdomen with organisms resistant to the antibiotic regimen he is receiving. Further antimicrobial administration and operative interventions are futile and may contribute to the peritoneal superinfection. The usually fatal outcome of tertiary peritonitis, which conceptually falls within the SIRS-MODS complex, indicates that current antibiotic-assisted, mechanical answers to severe peritonitis have about reached their limits, and the patient is rarely salvageable.

39 Anastomotic Leaks and Fistulas

"If there is a possibility of several things going wrong,
the one that will cause the most damage will be the one to go wrong"
(Arthur Bloch, Murphy's Law)

There are two chief clinical scenarios of postoperative intestinal leak:

- The leak is obvious – you see intestinal contents draining from the operative wound or from the drain site – if a drain was left.
- You suspect a leak but do not see one.

Scenario 1

It is postoperative day 6 after a laparotomy for small bowel obstruction (chapter 17) which was uneventful, except two accidental enterotomies – closed with an interrupted vicryl. During morning rounds the patient complains: "look, doctor, my bed is full with this green stuff ". You uncover the patient's abdomen – bile-stained intestinal juice is poring through the incision! Now you are very upset. True, the patient's recovery was not smooth; he was running a fever and a high white cell count; and now this terrible disaster!. It is a disaster indeed, for even today around one third of patients with intestinal suture-line breakdown die.

Your first reflex-thought is: "let's take him immediately to the operating room and fix up the mess". Is it advisable?

The Controversy

There is little controversy that established postoperative external enteocutaneous fistulas, which usually result from leaking anastomoses or incidental enterotomies, are to be treated initially *conservatively*. As noted in previous chapters, there is also little controversy that acute gastrointestinal perforation, be it spontaneous or traumatic, is an indication for an emergency laparotomy to deal with the source of contamination/infection (chapter 10).

So what about the "early postoperative small bowel leakage"? Is it a "simple perforation" – requiring an immediate operation, or a "fistula" to be managed conservatively? We contend that this scenario represent both conditions and should therefore be managed selectively in the individual patient.

The Role of Non-operative Management

With proper conservative-supportive management, and in the absence of distal obstruction or loss of bowel continuity, more than half of postoperative small bowel fistulas will close spontaneously. The remaining, which fail to close within six weeks, will require an elective re-operation. The latter, performed on an anabolic, non-SIRSing patient, in a less hostile peritoneal environment, will restore the gastrointestinal tract with a minimal rate of complications.

A crucial issue when deciding on a trial of conservative management is the absence or presence of peritonitis and/or "sepsis": clinical peritonitis is an indication for an immediate operation. Even when clinical peritonitis is not present, any evidence of "SIRS/SEPSIS" should promote an aggressive search for drainable intra-abdominal pus. This is best done with a CT scan: "associated" abscesses should be drained, percutaneously (PC) or at a laparotomy (chapter 35).

Remember: in unselected series of postoperative enteocutaneous fistulas a third of patients die – the vast majority from neglected intra-abdominal infection.

The Role of Operative Management

As stated above, peritonitis or a "complex" intra-abdominal abscess – not responding to PC drainage – is an indication for a laparotomy. But why not operate on all such patients? Why not just surrender to the temptation buzzing in your brain: "I know where this leak is coming from; let me just return to that abdomen and fix the small problem with a few more sutures". What should prevent you from re-suturing the leaking anastomosis or enterotomy?

Primary Closure of an Intestinal Suture Line Is Doomed to Fail

Each of you, and us, has had an isolated success in closing an intestinal leakage but the collective experience points to an overwhelmingly high rate of failure. Attempts to close an intestinal leak, after a few days, in an infected peritoneal cavity is doomed to fail; an intestinal anastomoses in the presence of postoperative peritonitis is an exercise in futility. Obviously, if successful the surgeon is a hero who saves his patient a prolonged hospitalization and morbidity. If, however, a leak re-develops, as it usually does, it represents a tremendous "second hit" – which strikes at an already primed, susceptible and compromised host (chapter 38). "Septic death" is then almost inevitable.

Suggested Approach to Early Postoperative Intestinal Fistula

Trial of conservative management is warranted when:
- There is no clinical peritonitis.
- There is no "associated" abscesses on CT.
- You know or can accurately guess the underlying cause of the leakage: you were the one to perform the first operation and know with a reasonable certainty where is the leakage originating from (an anastomosis or an enterotomy).

An immediate re-laparotomy is warranted when:
- Evidence of clinical peritonitis.

- " SIRS/Sepsis" with proven or suspected intra-peritoneal abscesses (PC attempt at drainage is in order, however).
- Abdominal compartment syndrome.
- Somebody you do not trust performed the primary, "index", operation. Bitter experience taught us that in such cases "anything is possible" and it is better to re-operate – you never know what the findings will be.

What To Do During an Emergency Re-laparotomy?

The decision is based on a few factors: 1. The condition of the bowel; 2. The condition of the peritoneal cavity; 3. The condition of the patient.

Very rarely: in a stable, minimally compromised patient, when peritonitis is macroscopically minimal, when the bowel appears of "good quality", when patient's serum albumin levels are reasonable – we would resect the involved segment and re-anastomose. Such a scenario is possible only when the leak presents within a day or two following the operation – usually caused by a technical mishap. An immediate re-operation before local and systemic adverse repercussions develop may thus provide definitive cure. Otherwise, the less heroic but logical and life saving option of exteriorization of the leaking point as an enterostomy should be carried out, and at *any level*.

Conservative Management

The principles of management are few and simple.
- *Restore fluid and electrolytes balance.* All fistula's losses should be replaced.
- *Protect the skin* around the fistula from the corrosive intestinal juice. A well fitting colostomy bag around the fistula's site often does the trick. Otherwise place a tube connected to a continuous

suction source at the fistula's site, place stomadhesive sheaths
around the defect, and cover the entire field with an adhesive
transparent dressing (similar to the "sandwich" described in chapter 37 but without the mesh).

- *Provide nutrition.* Proximal gastrointestinal fistula requires TPN.
  Distal small bowel and colonic fistulas will close spontaneously
  whether the patient is fed orally or not. As emphasized in chapter
  31, using the intestine if possible is better. In high fistula it is often
  possible, and beneficial, to collect the fistula's output, re-infusing
  it, together, with the enteral diet, into the bowel below the fistula.
- *Delineate anatomy.* This is best done with a sinogram – injecting
  water-soluble contrast into the fistula's tract: this will document
  the level of the bowel defect and the absence of distal obstruction
  and loss of continuity – perquisites for a successful conservative
  management.
- *Exclude and treat infection*: this has been mentioned above – and
  repeated here only to emphasize that when your fistula patient
  dies it is usually because you were not aggressive enough in
  pursuing our advice.

Gimmicks: the initial output of a fistula has little prognostic implications.
A fistula which drains 1000 ml per day during the first week has the same
chances to spontaneously seal as that with an output of 500 ml/ day.
Artificially decreasing fistula's output with total starvation and administration of somatostatin-analogue is cosmetically appealing but not proven
to be beneficial.

Fistula Associated with a Large Abdominal Wall Defect

Not uncommonly the end result of intestinal leaks and re-operative
surgery is an abdominal wall defect with multiple intestinal fistulas in its
base. *This so called "complex" or type IV fistula represents a catastrophe,*

346   *which carries a very high mortality rate.* (According to our classification
type A-are forgut fistulas; type B- small bowel; type C-colonic). The
distance of the fistulous opening in the intestine from the surface of the
defect and the condition of the peritoneal cavity has bearing on the
treatment of this condition. It is practical to distinguish between two
situations:

- *Type IV-A fistula*: when the fistula is located in the depth of the
  infected abdominal defect, the prolonged contact of large peritoneal
  surfaces with gastrointestinal contents allows increased absorption
  of toxic products, perpetuating local and systemic inflammatory
  response and organ dysfunction. In such instances re-operation is
  necessary to exteriorize or divert the intestinal leak away from the
  defect. Otherwise, the patient is doomed – more than half of the
  patients with this type of postoperative fistula die!

- *Type IV-B fistula*: those are "exposed" fistulas near the surface of
  the defect. Also called "bud" fistulas they result from damage to
  intestine exposed at the base of the defect. Because the peritoneal
  cavity is usually clean and sealed away from intestinal contents an
  expectant approach is indicated as early attempts at intestinal
  reconstruction are hazardous during the resolution of severe peritoneal inflammation. A simple rule of thumb is that the condition
  of the abdominal wall defect reflects the condition of the peritoneal cavity. A well contracted abdominal wall defect, and fistulas
  which look as surgical stomas are indicators that an elective intervention is possible and safe (chapter 37).

- Note: an "exposed-bud" fistula may be dealt temporarily (until
  definitive reconstruction) using the following technique: define the
  mucosal and submucosal layer of the pouting intestinal hole, close
  it with a fine monofilament suture. Immediately cover the repaired
  bowel and the surrounding abdominal wall defect with a split-
  thickness skin graft. This should be successful in half of your
  attempts.

Scenario 2:
You Suspect a Leak But Do Not See One

Your patient is now a week after an uneventful hemicolectomy for a carcinoma of the cecum. She is already at home, and eating, when a new pain develops at the right side of her abdomen, accompanied by vomiting. The patients return to the emergency room: she is febrile, her left abdomen is tender with a questionable mass, the abdominal X-ray suggests an ileus or partial small bowel obstruction (chapters 2 & 34). The white cell count is elevated. You suspect an anastomotic leak.

From a clinical standpoint there are three types of intestinal leaks that "you cannot see":

- *Free leak.* The anastomosis is disrupted and the leak is *not* contained by adjacent structures. The patients usually appear "sick", exhibiting signs of diffuse peritonitis. An immediate laparotomy is indicated as outlined above.
- *Contained leak.* The leak is partially contained by peri-anastomotic adhesions to the omentum and adjacent viscera. The clinical abdominal manifestations are *localized*. A peri-anastomotic abscess is a natural sequela.
- *A mini-leak.* This is a "minute" anastomotic leak – sually occurring late after the operation when the anastomosis is well sealed off. Abdominal manifestations are localized and the patient is not "toxic". A mini-leak is actually a "peri-anastomositis" – an inflammatory phlegmon around the anastomosis. Usually it is *not* associated with a dainable puss-containing abscess.

In the absence of diffuse peritonitis you should document the leak and grade it. Colonic anastomoses are best visualized with a gastrografin enema. For upper gastro-intestinal and small bowel anastomoses give gastrografin from above. We usually would combine the contrast study with a CT – searching for free intra-peritoneal contrast or abscesses.

348   There are a few possibilities:
- Free leak of contrast into the peritoneal cavity; a lot of free contrast and fluid on CT. You have to re-operate. We previously discussed what to do – best to take down the anastomosis.
- Contained localized leak, a local collection-abscess on CT. The rest of the peritoneal cavity is "dry". This is initially treated with antibiotics and PC drainage (chapter 35).
- No leak on contrast study, a peri-anastomotic phlegmon. This represents mini-leak or "peri-anastomositis" and usually resolves on a few days of antibiotic therapy.

Note that a contained leak or a mini-leak may be associated with an obstruction at the anastomosis – a result of the local inflammation. Such obstruction usually resolves spontaneously – within a week or so – after the pus has been drained and the inflammation has subsided.

Conclusion

We showed you that an anastomotic leak is not "one disease" but a wide spectrum of conditions requiring differential approaches. To keep morbidity at bay – tailor your treatment to the specific leak, it's degree and the affected patient. Above all – remember that non-drained intra-peritoneal bowel contents and pus are *killers* – often silent ones.

> **We tend to remember best those patients we almost killed;**
> **we never forget those we actually managed to kill**

40 Wound Management

The fate of the surgical wound is sealed during the operation;
almost nothing can be done after the operation
to modify the wound's outcome.

All that is visible to the patient of your wonderful, life saving, emergency abdominal operation is the surgical wound. Wound complications, although not life threatening are an irritating source of painful morbidity which bothers the patient and his surgeon alike. It is no wonder then that throughout generations, surgeons developed elaborate rituals to prevent and treat wound complications. Now, that you are reading the third to last chapter of this book you are, hopefully, sufficiently brain-washed to deplore elaborate gimmicks, and demand pragmatic solutions instead.

Definitions and the Spectrum

For practical purposes you do not need complicated definitions used by epidemiologists or infection-control nurses.

- An *uncomplicated* wound is a sutured wound that heals by primary intention and uneventfully. Note that following emergency abdominal surgery, an entirely uncomplicated wound is an exception! You do not believe us? Start to document from now on all your wounds and see for yourself the number of weeping or red-swollen wounds your patients have.
- *Complicated wounds.* Those are extremely common after emergency surgery when prospectively assessed by independent observers. Conversely, when "reported" by surgeons they become "rare" or "minor" – due to our natural tendency to suppress or ignore adverse outcome. The spectrum of wound complications is wide and encompasses infective and non-infective complications, minor and major.

• *Minor complications* are those irritating aberrations in the process
of healing which, however, do not impede primary healing of the
wound: a tiny hematoma, a little painful erythema, some serous
discharge. The distinction between an infectious and non-infectious
process is difficult and also unnecessary: why take swab-cultures
from such a wound if it would not affect therapy?

• *Major complications* are those which interfere with the process of
primary healing and require your intervention: large hematoma or
a wound abscess in need of drainage.

• *Wound infection*: for practical purposes this is a wound, which
contains pus that requires drainage. Usually such an infection represents a "walled-off" wound abscess, with minimal involvement of
adjacent soft tissues or underlying fascia. Rarely, surrounding
cellulitis is significant or the deep fascia is involved – denoting an
invasive infection.

Prevention

Surgical technique and overall patient care are of great importance in
minimizing the incidence of wound infection. Rarely is one aspect of
management of singular importance. It is the sum of the parts that yield
favorable results. The emergency nature of surgery you had to perform
is inherently associated with the contamination of the wound by intestinal
bacteria or by the established infections it treats (chapter 10). You also
do not have sufficient time to pre-operatively reverse all conditions,
which may add to the wound's risk such as shock, diabetes or malnutrition
(chapter 5). Although a certain rate of wound complications is "obligatory" –
inherent in the nature of this type of surgery – you should strive to keep
it as low as possible. How?

Let us reiterate here the above-mentioned aphorism: "*The fate of
the surgical wound is sealed during the operation; almost nothing can be*

done after the operation to modify the wound's outcome". Whether your   351
patient develops a wound hematoma or infection depends on your patient
and on you, and is determined during the operation – not afterwards.

Meticulous technique as described in chapter 29 is paramount.
Here a few preventive points are re-emphasized:

- Operate fast and carefully – not masturbating the tissues.
- Do not strangulate the fascia with interrupted – figure of eight
  sutures of wire, ethibond or vicryl – use instead low-tension
  continuous spring like monofilament closure – letting the abdominal
  wall breath (chapter 29).
- Do not charcoal the skin and underlying tissues with excessive use
  of diathermy.
- Do not bury tons of highly irritating chromic in the subcutaneous
  fat.
- Do not close skin with the even more irritating silk.
- Do not exit contaminating colostomies through the main abdominal
  wound.
- Do not leave useless drains in the wound.

Antibiotics

Antibiotic prophylaxis reduces the wound infection rate; its anti-infective
effects are in fact more pronounced in the surgical wound than within
the peritoneal cavity (chapter 6). Intra-incisional antibiotics have also
a preventive role (chapter 29); this makes sense if you consider that the
wound's defense mechanisms are much weaker than that of the peritoneal
cavity. Many years ago it has been shown that antibiotics are effective in
preventing wound infections only if given within 3 hours of bacterial
contamination – the "effective period". *Postoperative antibiotics cannot
change the fate of the wound*! Despite what you have been told hitherto
by your local infectious disease specialists, an adequate peri-operative

352   antibiotic coverage is as effective in preventing wound infection as 7 days of administration (chapter 32).

Non-closure or Delayed Closure of the Wound

Leaving the skin and subcutis completely or partially open following contaminated or "dirty" procedures is still advocated by some "authorities". True; it may prevent wound infections in the minority of patients which are bound to develop one. At the same time leaving all wounds open condemns the majority – whose wounds are destined to heal uneventfully – to the morbidity of open wounds, it's management, and the risk of superinfection. For more details about this controversial issue look at chapter 29.

Management-the Uncomplicated Wound

The uncomplicated primarily closed surgical wound needs almost no care. A day after the operation it is well sealed away from the external environment by a layer of fibrin. It can be left exposed. Isn't it ridiculous to see gloved and masked nurses changing sterile dressings on routine surgical wounds? Some patients demand their wounds to be covered; cheap dry gauze is more than adequate for this purpose. The chief aim of elaborate "modern" dressing material is to enrich the medical-industrial complex. Patients with uncomplicated wounds can shower or bath any time.

Management – the Complicated Wound   353

Here the punishment should fit the crime. Minor "non specific" complications should be observed – the majority will resolve spontaneously.
Again, starting antibiotics because a wound "weeps" a little serous
discharge is not going to change anything; if the wound is destined to
develop an infection it will – with or without antibiotics! Major wound
hematomas require evacuation but this is extremely rare following
abdominal surgery.

Management of Wound Infections.

Wound infection following emergency abdominal operation is caused
usually by endogenous bacteria – the resident bacteria of the abdominal
organs breached during the operation or the bacteria which caused the
intra-abdominal infection. Following non-contaminated operations
(e.g. blunt splenic trauma) the bugs causing wound infections are exoge-
nous – skin residents, usually a *Staph*.

   A *Strep* wound cellulitis may develop a day after the operation with
pain, swelling and erythema and elevated temperature, but we have
never seen one. Wound infections also may present in your private office
even weeks after the operation – skewing your hospital infection-control
data. When in doubt, do not rush to poke in or open the wound – creating
complications in wounds that would otherwise heal. Instead, be patient,
wait a day or two – let the infection "mature" and declare itself.

   As a rule: removing a few skin sutures and draining the pus treats
most wound infections. Aftercare should be simple: shallow wounds are
covered with dry gauze and cleaned twice daily with water and soap – there
is nothing better for an open wound than a shower or bath! Deeper
wounds are *loosely* packed with gauze to afford drainage and prevent
premature closure of the superficial layers. Antibiotics are not necessary.

354   Do you give antibiotics after the incision and drainage of a peri-anal abscess? Of course not. So why treat wound infections with antibiotics? A short course of antimicrobials is indicated when severe cellulitis is present or the abdominal fascia is involved (i.e. invasive infection).

Wound swabs; wound cultures; Gram stains? What for? As you know by now, the causative bacteria are predictable (chapter 10) and beside how could the microbiological results change the therapy outlined above?

Nurses and for-profit home care agencies push forward elaborate and expensive wound care methods in order to justify their continued involvement. Local application of solutions or ointments of antiseptics or antibiotics destroy microorganisms and human cells alike, induce allergy and induce bacterial resistance. *Expensive forms of wound coverage are a gimmick. Simple is beautiful.*

Minor complication is one that happens to somebody else.

41 The Role of Laparoscopy

The world might look brighter through
the (laparoscopic) camera – but not everything bright is gold

Laparoscopic options were mentioned 'en passe' in the preceding chapters but a promise was made to further elaborate on the role of laparoscopy in abdominal emergencies. To do so we had to summon help from a surgeon who is more enthusiastic than us. Here it goes:

Diagnostic laparoscopy was used for many decades by gynecologists to investigate acute pelvic disorders. With the recent boom in basic and advanced laparoscopic techniques no wonder that enthusiasts started to explore the role of laparoscopy in the diagnosis and treatment of almost any abdominal emergency. The rational is simple: laparoscopy may offer an organ-specific diagnosis and at the same time provide treatment-avoiding a laparotomy. This could minimize morbidity and patient's discomfort, shortens hospital stay, accelerate recovery, and improve patients' satisfaction.

Laparoscopy has been used both in acute non-traumatic and traumatic abdominal situations. Master-laparoscopists – great aficiona-dos – claim to be able to do "anything" through the laparoscope. Dour conservationists, on the other hand, almost totally reject laparoscopy, except perhaps for very selected indications – such as acute cholecystitis (chapter 15), acute appendicitis (chapter 22), gynecological emergencies (chapter 25) and left thoraco-abdominal trauma (chapter 26). The following, we hope, is an enlightened – modern but balanced – view.

Non-traumatic Abdominal Pain

Let us start emphasizing that *laparoscopy* is absolutely *contra-indicated in* critically ill *hemodynamically unstable* patients. Just face it: laparoscopy takes more time, and in severely compromised patients you want to find the source of the problem and deal with it as fast as possible. In addition, that pneumoperitoneum elevates intra-abdominal pressure, which is deleterious in unstable, 'septic', and ill patients, was discussed above (chapter 28). A sure way to produce a cardiac arrest is to take a hypovolemic patient, anesthetize him, and then pump up his abdomen with gas (CO_2).

Laparoscopy can be performed as a part of diagnostic process, as a therapeutic procedure or both. Its application and availability largely depends on surgeon's experience and prompt access to laparoscopic instrumentation. Diagnostic laparoscopy (DL) can be performed expeditiously and even outside the operating room – in the emergency room or SICU – and under local anesthesia. The morbidity from negative DL, as compared to negative or non-therapeutic laparotomy, is lower. The use of mini-laparoscopy (instruments smaller than 3 mm in diameter) is gaining popularity and may further diminish the invasiveness of the procedure.

DL assesses the presence and amount of intra-peritoneal blood, bowel contents, or pus, and establishes its source. A decision is then made whether control of the source is necessary, and if yes – should it be performed laparoscopically or through a laparotomy.

Clinical Conditions Commonly Approached Laparoscopically

- Diagnosis of the abdominal pain with equivocal physical examination and abdominal imaging (chapter 3)

- Acutely perforated peptic ulcer (chapter 13)   357
- Acute cholecystitis (chapter 15)
- Acute appendicitis (chapter 22)
- Acute gynecological pathology, such as PID, ruptured ovarian cyst, ectopic pregnancy (chapter 25)

Controversial Application of Laparoscopy

- Bleeding peptic ulcer (chapter 12)
- Intestinal obstruction (chapter 17)
- Intestinal ischemia (chapter 19)
- Acute diverticulitis (chapter 23)
- Acute abdomen in pregnant patient (chapter 25)

Balancing Comment

The role of laparoscopy in the diagnosis and treatment of non-traumatic abdominal emergencies is evolving. Hitherto, it has it reached wide acceptance in acute cholecystitis and gynecological conditions. There is a strong rational to embark on laparoscopy when the source of right lower quadrant pain is questionable – especially in a female patient. Many surgeons favor laparoscopic appendectomy but its benefits are marginal. It appears that when the appendix is perforated-"septic", intra-abdominal complications are lesser with the open technique. In addition 'lap-appy' is attractive in the very obese patient. In order to be able and confident to tackle other conditions through the laparoscope you must be able to laparoscopically explore the various spaces and corners of the peritoneal cavity. You have to be skilled in advanced laparoscopic techniques and intracorporeal suturing techniques if you wish to deal laparoscopically with more complicated situations such as perforated peptic ulcer.

358   *Remember*: the acutely ill patient is not a suitable guinea pig for your budding laparoscopic ambitions. The sicker the patient, the more diffuse is his peritonitis – the less suitable candidate he is for your magic lenses and trocars. Be selective and balanced.

Laparoscopy for Abdominal Trauma

You may remember that in chapters 26 & 27 we were quite skeptical about the role of laparoscopy in the trauma patient. Let us hear, however, what the enthusiast has to sell:

Blunt Trauma

Management decisions in blunt abdominal trauma are based on the patient's hemodynamic status and physical findings, and the selective and complementary use of diagnostic ultrasonography, CT, and diagnostic peritoneal lavage (DPL). So what is the place of laparoscopy?

Its main role is to further avoid non-therapeutic laparotomies, this decreasing postoperative morbidity and hospital stay. But, first, again- the contraindications: *laparoscopy should be performed only in hemodynamically stable patient with no urgent indication for laparotomy*.

The good candidate for DL is a stable patient with equivocal findings on physical examination, CT or DPL. DL can achieve organ specific diagnosis, identify and quantify the presence of peritoneal blood, bile or intestinal content, grade the severity of injury to the liver and spleen, assess whether there is active bleeding and its rate, and rule out diaphragmatic injury. In selected patients, with minimal injury, laparoscopy may become therapeutic – for example – evacuating blood, and achieving hemostasis of a small hepatic tear.

Penetrating Trauma

Stab wounds: patients with clinical indications for a laparotomy, i.e. peritonitis or shock, are managed with an immediate laparotomy. DL has a potential role when clinical findings are equivocal, and especially in thoracoabdominal wounds – to rule out diaphragmatic penetration. Laparoscopy may become therapeutic when injury is minimal.

Gunshot wounds (GSW): The vast majority of the GSW are managed with an immediate laparotomy. Only a minority of patients with stable vital signs and no peritonitis are candidates for DL to exclude abdominal penetration or prove that the injury is minimal and does not require a laparotomy. Again, with thoracoabdominal GSW diaphragmatic injury has to be excluded.

Balancing Comment

'Selective conservatism' based on clinical assessment (chapter 26) is a well-tested, safe and cheap approach in patients with stab wounds to the abdomen. The advantages of performing invasive DL in such patients is unsubstantiated and difficult to justify. True, DL is the most sensitive method to diagnose an "occult" penetration of the left diaphragm – which is commonly associated with left thoracoabdominal wounds, but the natural history of this entity – if left untreated – is unknown. With GSW, 'selective conservatism' is also possible in the minority of patients but adopted reluctantly by surgeons. Here, in stable patients with borderline abdominal signs, DL may prove that the GSW was extra-peritoneal-tangential. A crucial limitation of laparoscopy is that it cannot adequately assess retroperitoneal structures such as the colon, duodenum, kidneys and vessels. It confirms or excludes peritoneal penetration but in terms of assessing the damage a CT is more sensitive and less invasive. Be aware of the risk of tension pneumothorax when performing a DL in patient

360   with diaphragmatic penetration. Deflating the pneumoperitoneum and the insertion of a chest tube can reverse it. Gas embolism is a potential complication when major venous injuries are present but as our expert points out – it has never been reported in thousands of cases. It appears that the role of laparoscopy in the injured patient is limited, but laparoscopic aficionados claim that growing experience and developing instrumentation will expand its role in the future.

Advanced tools in the hands of fools are not cool

42 In the Aftermath
and the M & M Meeting

"Big" operation in "fit" patients may be "small"
"Small" operation in sick patients may be "big"
A "big" surgeon knows to tailor the operation
and its trauma to the patient and his disease

Again and again I find that there are few things so quickly forgotten
by the surgical system as a dead patient
(PO Nystrom)

Let us hope that your patient survives his emergency abdominal operation and his postoperative course is uneventful. Unfortunately, the overall mortality of such procedures is still far from negligible and the morbidly rate is generally high. Now, after the storm has waned, it is the time to sit down and reflect on what went wrong.

The Mortality & Morbidly Meeting

At any place where a group of surgeons is working it is crucial to conduct a regular M & M Meeting (MMM). This is the venue where you and your colleagues should *objectively* analyze and discuss – in retrospect – all the recent moralities and complications. You are familiar with the cliché' that 'some surgeons learn from their own mistakes, some learn from that of others, and some never learn'. The aim of the MMM is to abolish the latter entity.

Do you have a regular M & M meeting in your Department? If you are associated, as a resident or a qualified surgeon, with a teaching Department in the USA, you must have a weekly MMM, because without

362   a routine MMM the Department's residency program cannot be accredited. We know that in many corners around the world MMM are not conducted – all blunders and failures are buried below the carpet. Elsewhere still, MMM exist only in name – being used to present "interesting cases' or the last "stories of success". This is wrong. MMM exist to objectively analyze your mistakes and complications – not to punish or humiliate anyone, but to educate and improve results. You do not want to repeat the same error twice. See to it that proper MMM's are conducted wherever you provide surgical care.

Format of the MMM

- A routine hour should be dedicated to the MMM each week.
- ALL interns, residents and surgeons should attend – regularly.
- ALL complications and deaths, which occurred in any patient treated by any member of the Department should be presented.
- 'Complication is a complication' – irrespective whether the outcome was a triumph or tragedy. All must be presented.
- The MMM is a democratic forum. The Boss's blunder or that by the "local giant" is as "interesting", if not more so, as that caused by a junior resident.

The resident-team, which was involved with the case, should present it. They should know all details and rehearse the presentation in advance. The patient's chart and X rays should be readily available. If you are the presenting resident be objective and neutral. Your task is to learn and facilitate learning of others – not to "defend" or "cover up" the involved surgeon – you are not his or her lawyer. Understand that the majority of those who are present are not stupid – they sense immediately when truth is deserted.

The Assessment of Complications   363

After the case has been presented the person who presides over the meeting has to initiate and generate a discussion with the intent to arrive at a consensus. An easy way to break the commonly prevailing and embarrassing silence is to point at one of the senior surgeons and ask: "Dr. X, please tell us, had this patient been under *your* care from the beginning – would the outcome be the same?" This technique usually manages to break the ice, prompting a sincere and complete response.

The questions to be answered during the discussion are:

- *Was it a "real complication"?* Some surgeons may argue that a blood loss, which required transfusion, is not a "complication" but a "technical mishap" – which simply "can happen".
- *Assess the cause*: was it an error in *judgement* or a *technical* error? Operating on a dying terminal cancer patient reflects poor judgement; having to re-operate for hemorrhage from the gallbladder's bed marks a technical error – poor hemostasis at the first operation. *The two types of errors are often combined and inseparable*: the patient with acute bowel ischemia died because his operation was "too late" (poor judgement) and the stoma, which was performed, has retracted, leaking into the peritoneal cavity (poor technique). Often it is impossible to define whether a "technical complication"- e.g. anastomotic leak – is caused by poor technique (technical error) or "patient's related" factors, such as malnutrition or steroid intake.
- Another possibility is to look at the error as either an error of *commission* or *omission*. One either operates too late or not at all (*omission*) or operates too early or unnecessarily (*commission*). One either misses the injury or resects" too little" (*omission*) or does "too much" (*commission*). After the operation one either fails to re-operate for the abscess (*omission*) or operates unnecessarily – when percutaneous drainage was possible (*commission*). Note that the surgical community considers errors of omission more gravely

that those of commission; the latter are looked at with understanding: "we did all what we can but we failed".

- *Was there negligence? A certain rate of mistakes (hopefully low) is a integral part of any surgical practice as only those who never operate commit no errors, but negligence is deplorable.* The operation was delayed because the responsible surgeon did not want to be disturbed over the weekend or the surgeon operated under influence of alcohol: this is clearly "negligence". When an individual surgeon repeats errors over and over again – a paradigm is exhibited, which in itself may constitute a "negligence".

- *Was the complication/death preventable or potentially preventable?* We encourage our residents to report the physiologic score of acute disease-APACHE II (chapter 5) of the presented patient. Low pre-operative scores (< 10) means that the patient's predicted operative mortality was very low, suggesting a preventable death such as anesthetic mishap. A very high score (>20) does not imply however that the patient was unsalvageable. High-risk patients are those who require superb judgement and technical skills; these are the patients who do not tolerate even the smallest error.

- *Who was responsible?* The MMM is not a court. But at the end of the presentation it should be clear to all present whose culprit it was. Can we toss the responsibility on the anesthetist who extubated the patient too early, on the resident who misplaced the endotracheal tube in the esophagus, or must we take the responsibility on ourselves?

- *Was the standard of care met?* As you surely know, the "standard of care" means different things to different people. It has a spectrum, which should be well represented and assessed by a group of well-informed practicing surgeons. Take, for example, a case of perforated sigmoid diverticulitis with local peritonitis (chapter 23); any operation ranging from a Hartmann's procedure (the conservative surgeon) to a sigmoid resection with anastomosis (the modern

surgeon) would fall within the accepted standard of care. Primary   365
closure of the perforation would not. Easy to assess: "anyone who
would attempt closing the perforation please raise his hand". No
hand is raised; the responsible surgeon is left lonely to understand
that what he did is not acceptable; it is outside the practiced
standard *in his community*. The responsible surgeon may however
present published literature to support that what he did is acceptable elsewhere.

- *Evidence based surgery*. At the end of the presentation the resident
  should present literature to pinpoint the "state of the art" and the
  associated controversies, emphasizing "what could have been done,
  and should be done when we see a similar case in the future".
- *The surgeon who is responsible for the complication*. At the end of
  the discussion the most senior surgeon involved in the care of the
  concerned patient should offer a statement. He may chose to present
  additional evidence from the published literature to show that what
  he did is acceptable elsewhere. The most graceful way to deal with
  the situation is to frankly discuss the case scenario and humbly
  admit the mistakes one has committed. If you had another chance
  with the same patient how would you manage him? By standing up
  and "confessing" you gain the respect of all present. When you lie,
  cover-up, not accepting the "verdict" of the gathering, you evoke silent contempt and resentment. So stand up and admit!

Conclusions and Corrective Measures

Finally the person in chair has to conclude: was it an error? Whose fault
was it? Was the standard of care met? And what are the future recommendations and the corrective measures? If you are that chairperson,
and you may be some day – don't be wishy-washy. Be objective and
"definitive" for the audience is not stupid.

Financial Morbidity

In this day and age of growing costs and limited resources we must not
ignore the *financial morbidity*: the excessive spending on unnecessary
procedures, even if the later were not associated with an immediately-
visible physical morbidity. When discussing the case, ask the presenter to
justify the Swan Ganz catheter which has been inserted, or what was the
reason to continue antibiotics for seven days; or why was the patient
"observed" in the SICU after an uneventful laparotomy? A useful educa-
tional exercise is to randomly present a detailed summary of the hospital
bill of a presented patient. Knowing how much things cost and what is
the financial prize of your superfluous acts, and how much the complications you created – actually cost in $ US or Euro, will make you a more
careful surgeon.

The SURGINET

An "ideal" and objective MMM as featured above is not conducted in
many places because of local sociopolitical restrains. If this is the case in
your neck of the woods, it may be damaging to your own surgical education: how would you know what is right or wrong? Books and journals
are useful but cannot replace a thorough analysis of specific cases by a
group of leaned surgeons. Well, if you have a PC and an e-mail access
you can subscribe to SURGINET-an international forum of surgeons,
who would openly and objectively discuss any case or complication you
present to them. Should you want to take part in this "international
MMM" send an e-mail message to
Dr. Tom Gilas of Toronto: *tgilas@sympatico.ca*
or to the editor of this book: *mschein1@mindspring.com.*

Conclusions

367

As you know – there are many ways to skin a cat, and it is easy to be a smart-ass – looking at things through the "retroscope". Our sick patients and the events leading to the MMM are very complex. But behind all this complex chaos there is always an eternal truth – which should be and can be disclosed and announced. As Winston Churchill said: *success is "the ability to go from failure to failure without losing your enthusiasm."*

Failure obliges change-success breeds complacency

Subject Index

Printed in Italy by Legoprint S.p.A., Lavis (Trento)